D1228349

JOSEPH I. ROUTH, Ph.D.

Professor, Department of Biochemistry, College
of Medicine, The University of Iowa, Iowa City, Iowa

Mathematical Preparation for the Health Sciences

Second Edition

WITHDRAWN FROM
WILLIAM F. MAAG LIBRARY
YOUNGSTOWN STATE UNIVERSITY

1976

W. B. SAUNDERS COMPANY

Philadelphia, London, Toronto

W. B. Saunders Company: West Washington Square
Philadelphia, PA 19105

1 St. Anne's Road
Eastbourne, East Sussex BN21 3UN, England

833 Oxford Street
Toronto, Ontario M8Z 5T9, Canada

Library of Congress Cataloging in Publication Data

Routh, Joseph Isaac, 1910-

Mathematical Preparation for the Health Sciences

First ed. published in 1971 under title: Mathematical Preparation
for Laboratory Technicians.

1. Medicine – Mathematics. I. Title.

RB 38.2.R68 1976   616.07'56'0151   75-25274

ISBN   0-7216-7736-3

Mathematical Preparation for the Health Sciences   ISBN 0–7216–7736–3

© 1976 by W. B. Saunders Company. Copyright 1971 by W. B. Saunders Company. Copyright under the International Copyright Union. All rights reserved. This is
protected by copyright. No part of it may be reproduced, stored in a retrieval system, or
transmitted in any form or by any means, electronic, mechanical, photocopying, recording
or otherwise, without written permission from the publisher. Made in the United States of
America. Press of W. B. Saunders Company. Library of Congress catalog card number
75–25274.

Last digit is the print number: 9   8   7   6   5   4   3   2   1

2B
38.2
R68
976

PREFACE
TO THE
SECOND EDITION

For many years the author has been convinced of the need for a book that would assist a student in applying his mathematical knowledge to the solution of practical laboratory problems. The majority of students have confidence in their ability to carry out the common mathematical manipulations required to solve problems in addition, subtraction, multiplication, and division. The shortcomings so frequently observed in a scientific discipline or laboratory are the inability to apply these skills to a practical problem and the failure to recognize as correct or incorrect the answer that is the end result of the student's efforts.

Hopefully, the first edition of this book was a start in the right direction, and the many favorable comments and constructive criticisms received by the author were sincerely appreciated. The encouraging response has resulted in the present second edition, in which extensive changes and additions have been incorporated.

Since mathematical material for radiologic technologists and nuclear medical technologists has been added to this edition, the order of the presentation of the contents has been changed. Material common to all laboratory specialties is covered in the early chapters, including chapters on handling numbers, logarithms, the slide rule, concentration of solutions, hydrogen ion concentration and pH, and buffers. More specialized topics such as renal clearance calculations and spectrophotometric calculations follow these chapters. A new chapter on radiologic calculations is followed by chapters on the preparation of graphs and quality control statistics.

In the early chapters new material on the handling of fractions has been added, along with new worked-out examples in the chapters on the concentration of solutions and buffers. The system of S.I. units has been explained and incorporated into the problems in the book. The last three chapters include explanations and examples of calculations commonly encountered in nuclear medical technology, with graphical solutions in this field supplementing the material on the preparation of graphs and quality control material pertinent to nuclear medicine. Several new items have been included in the Appendix to

iii

WILLIAM F. MAAG LIBRARY
YOUNGSTOWN STATE UNIVERSITY
381161

make this section more informative. A new table of logarithms, a table of antilogarithms, material on the normality of concentrated solutions of acids and bases, a nomogram for acid-base balance and pCO_2, two nomograms for body surface area calculations, a radioactive decay table for ^{125}I, and a table of t values for the t test have been added to the Appendix. As in the first edition, answers for all exercises are included in the Appendix.

The author is deeply indebted to all the students, laboratory technicians, and instructors who submitted comments and constructive criticisms of the material in the first edition. Special appreciation is extended to Robert La Due and Glenn Isserstedt, who reviewed and criticized the material for nuclear medical technologists. The efforts of Linda Brown and Gene Putz, who evaluated the manuscript prior to publication, are greatly appreciated. Lynn Stoll deserves special thanks for her assistance in the preparation and typing of the manuscript and her continuing efforts to improve the book.

Finally the author is pleased to acknowledge the assistance of the editors and production staff of the W. B. Saunders Company, particularly Brian Decker, whose ideas and plans for improvement are incorporated in this second edition.

JOSEPH I. ROUTH

WILLIAM F. MAAG LIBRARY
YOUNGSTOWN STATE UNIVERSITY
351184

PREFACE
TO THE
FIRST EDITION

The majority of students have been exposed to a mathematics course every year throughout grade school, junior high, senior high and often in college. This extensive diet of arithmetic, algebra, plane and solid geometry, trigonometry and sometimes differential and integral calculus should result in a large number of mathematically oriented students. It would appear that students electing to specialize in some branch of chemistry or in a health-related science such as medical technology, pharmacy, dentistry or medicine should have achieved a firm foundation in mathematics and the ability to apply it to their specialty.

The author's contention, based on over three decades of teaching experience with students in the aforementioned disciplines, is that the multiple mathematics course system has not achieved a practical goal. It is obvious that all these courses are not required to prepare a student to add, subtract, multiply or divide properly. Algebraic, geometric and trigonometric functions are often memorized but seldom applied to practical situations. Unfortunately the meaningful application of mathematics often awaits the choice of a professional career. Long after the great mass of equations, theorems and exercises is forgotten the student is suddenly faced with the unfamiliar mathematical requirements of a scientific specialty.

At the risk of insulting the intelligence of mathematically oriented students this book stresses arithmetical common sense. In a classic sense it is not truly a mathematics book, but rather a book that reviews techniques in mathematics and applies these techniques to the solution of practical problems in a chemistry or health science laboratory.

The first three chapters set the stage for the application of mathematics in the laboratory. The material is obviously a review for many students and hopefully presents a practical foundation for techniques of problem solving in later chapters. If adequate time is spent considering the explanations and working the problems in these chapters, the subsequent material will be much easier to understand. Chapter 4 considers laboratory problems in the preparation of solutions, expressions of concentration, conversion from one type of concentration unit to another and dilution problems that commonly occur in the laboratory. The preparation of graphs, the substance of Chapter 5, often poses a difficult problem for laboratory technicians faced with calibration, standard curves, or kinetic measurements. Calculations involving spectrophotometric measurements are considered in Chapter 6, followed by the application of elementary statistics to quality control programs in Chapter 7. Chapters 8 and 9 cover the practical application of calculations involving pH and hydrogen ion concentration and buffer solutions to the preparation of buffers and the subject of acid-base balance. The final chapter is concerned with explanations of renal clearance test calculations.

To enable the student to check his understanding of the application of the material to the solution of problems and exercises in the book, answers for each exercise are given in the Appendix.

The author is indebted to so many students, instructors and laboratory technicians for their questions, problems and discussions that it would be most difficult to thank specific individuals for their role in the conception of the book. Susan Kracht deserves special thanks for her assistance in the preparation and typing of the manuscript. Grateful appreciation is due all of the instructors who criticized the manuscript prior to publication, including Sister Elizabeth Kramer, John Abadi, Carla Salmon, Jan Platt, Wayne Patton and Martha Olliver. Most important is the opportunity to express loving thanks to my wife Dorothy for her constant encouragement and insistence that the book would help present and future technicians. Finally the author is pleased to acknowledge the continual assistance of the editors and production staff of the W. B. Saunders Company.

JOSEPH I. ROUTH

CONTENTS

Simple Mathematical Manipulations

THE *PRACTICAL OBJECTIVES* OF THIS CHAPTER ARE TO OBTAIN AN UNDERSTANDING OF:

1. Arithmetical common sense.

2. The conversion of centigrade to Fahrenheit and Fahrenheit to centigrade temperatures.

3. The powers of ten and their application.

4. The use of fractions and their decimal equivalents.

As a positive approach to our cooperative efforts it may help to state that this is not a math book. To repeat, this is not a mathematics book, but rather a book that reviews techniques in mathematics and applies these techniques to the solution of practical problems in the laboratory. You have had over ten years of schooling in mathematical principles, have been taught repeatedly how to add, subtract, multiply, and divide, memorized geometric and trigonometric functions, and possibly mastered the use of logarithms. Yet laboratory calculations and problems of a practical nature often seem confusing and beyond reach of your knowledge. The major problem always seems to be a lack of confidence in the correctness of the answer you obtain when performing calculations of a practical nature. Overmemorization of principles and short-term memorization to pass an exam are major reasons for impractical knowledge of mathematics.

If a small fraction of your mental effort had been spent on **arithmetical common sense** your laboratory calculations would seem less formidable. With the mathematical background possessed by most students it is not too difficult to achieve arithmetical common sense. This is the ability to reason out a problem, to make sense out of the values used in multiplication and division and most of all to obtain a correct answer and to know that it is correct. Many people marvel at the ability of a person to figure out problems in his head. There is obviously nothing magical involved but merely an orderly process of making sense out of the manipulations required to solve a problem and occasionally being able to mentally calculate the exact values. This process is not essential to arithmetical common sense but is often quite dramatic. It is sufficient to be able to think through the problem in terms of rounded off values and come up with a sensible approximate answer.

Let us start with some very simple examples and work our way into laboratory mathematics. Problems involving the English system, rather than the metric system, of measurement may serve as a good start. If someone asked you how many feet there were in a yard or how many inches in a foot, you would automatically remember 3 feet to the yard and 12 inches to the foot. You may not remember how many yards there are in a mile, but if you were told that there were 5280 feet in a mile, you could probably work out in your head the number of yards per mile. Your mental gymnastics might operate as follows:

> I know there are 3 feet in a yard, so 5280 divided by 3 would equal 1 with 2 to carry, and 3 goes into 22 seven times with 1 to carry, and 18 divided by 3 is 6; so if I remember correctly, the answer would be 1760 yards in a mile.

It would not make sense to estimate 176 as an answer since 3 times 176 would not come close to 5280. This is a simple example of working a problem in your head and making sense out of the answer.

The unit of weight in the metric system is the kilogram, although 1/1000 of a kilogram, called a gram, is a very common measure of weight. In the laboratory many methods involve milligrams, which are 1/1000 of a gram, or micrograms, 1/1000 of a milligram. The conversion of these units is not too difficult to master mentally. Yet in the supermarkets many items are sold by the pound, and even people are still commonly weighed in pounds. If you are told that a kilogram equals approximately 2.2 pounds, how could you use this value to convert pounds to kilograms, pounds to grams and kilograms to pounds? Again, you reason that it takes over 2 lb to make 1 kg, so a 150 pound person is going to weigh less than one-half that value in kilograms, or less than 75 kg. In fact, 150 divided by 2.2 is about 68 kg. It still sounds more interesting to hear that a beauty queen tips the scales at 110 lb rather than 50 kg. Chemicals are often sold in 1 lb or 5 lb bottles, yet we use the chemicals in grams. From our original approximation of 1 kg equals 2.2 lb we can state that 1000 g equals 2.2 lb or 1 lb equals approximately 450 g.

In conversion problems it is sometimes difficult to avoid the use of memorized formulas or equations. This becomes clear if we examine the common centigrade and Fahrenheit temperature scales. The centigrade scale is often referred to as the Celsius scale, and degrees on the centigrade scale are termed degrees Celsius. We will use degrees C ($^\circ$C) as degrees centigrade since this is relevant to the explanation of the basis of the scale that follows. The centigrade scale was designed to make the freezing point of water read 0°C and the boiling point read 100°C, giving rise to the name "centigrade." The Fahrenheit scale reads 32°F at the freezing point and 212°F at the boiling point of water. Between the freezing and boiling points of water there are 100 centigrade and 180 Fahrenheit intervals or degrees; therefore, 100 centigrade intervals equal 180 Fahrenheit intervals. From this we conclude that

$$1° \text{ centigrade} = \frac{180}{100} = \frac{9°}{5} \text{ Fahrenheit}$$

and

$$1° \text{ Fahrenheit} = \frac{100}{180} = \frac{5°}{9} \text{ centigrade}$$

Even though the freezing point of water is 0° centigrade and 32° Fahrenheit, the temperature reads the same on both scales at – 40°. The simplest equations for the conversion of °C to °F or °F to °C are based on the 9/5 and 5/9 relationship and the value 40. In either case add 40 to the original temperature, multiply by either 5/9 or 9/5 and subtract 40 from the result. To decide which fraction to use it helps to choose a common point like the boiling point of water, 212°F and 100°C. It can readily be seen that the Fahrenheit value is higher than the centigrade value; therefore you would use the largest fraction, 9/5, to convert centigrade to Fahrenheit. The following examples may help illustrate the point.

Examples

To convert 100°C to Fahrenheit add 40, 100 + 40 = 140.
Multiply by $\frac{9}{5}$, $140 \times \frac{9}{5} = 252$.
Subtract 40, 252 – 40 = 212°F.

Or in outline form to convert 32°F to degrees centigrade:

$$32°F + 40 = 72$$
$$72 \times \frac{5}{9} = \frac{360}{9} = 40$$
$$40 – 40 = 0°C$$

Conversion of values below zero requires a sensible approach to the algebraic sum of the signs. To convert – 15°F to degrees centigrade:

$$-15°F + 40 = +25$$
$$+25 \times \frac{5}{9} = \frac{125}{9} = +14$$
$$+14 – 40 = -26°C$$

1.1 HANDLING NUMBERS

Numbers are very useful; in fact, they are essential in science courses and in the laboratory. A knowledge of the simplest way to handle numbers is obviously an asset in calculations. In general we should always express numbers in a form that can be readily used and equally readily understood. A uniform practice having many advantages is to express a large or small number as an integer (a number between 1 and 10) multiplied by a power of ten. As examples: $1000 = 1.0 \times 10^3$; $50,000 = 5 \times 10^4$; $0.001 = 10^{-3}$ and $0.000062 = 6.2 \times 10^{-5}$. If you count the number of zeros required to move a decimal point to obtain a number between 1 and 10 in the first two examples, you will obtain the correct positive power of ten.

Examples

$$1_\wedge000 = 1 \times 10^3 \qquad 5_\wedge0000 = 5 \times 10^4$$
$$321 \qquad\qquad 4321$$

The same scheme may be applied to large, more complex numbers such as 135,000 and 2467.

$$1_\wedge35000 = 1.35 \times 10^5 \qquad 2_\wedge467 = 2.467 \times 10^3$$
$$54321 \qquad\qquad\qquad 321$$

In numbers less than one, if you count the number of zeros and the first whole number, you have to move the decimal point to obtain a number between 1 and 10; the correct negative power of ten is thus obtained.

$$0.001_\wedge = 1 \times 10^{-3} \qquad 0.00006_\wedge2 = 6.2 \times 10^{-5}$$
$$123 \qquad\qquad\qquad 12345$$

Further examples of negative powers of ten are:

$$0.0001_\wedge46 = 1.46 \times 10^{-4} \qquad 0.0000007_\wedge34 = 7.34 \times 10^{-7}$$
$$1234 \qquad\qquad\qquad\qquad 1234567$$

Since, as will be seen in Chapters 2 and 3, the exponent of ten is identical with the characteristic of the corresponding logarithm of a number, the use of logarithms or a slide rule is simplified.

To multiply numbers expressed as powers of ten, first multiply the numbers (between 1 and 10) that are on the left of 10 to the power, then add the powers of ten.

$$200,000 \times 3,000,000 = 2 \times 10^5 \times 3 \times 10^6 = 2 \times 3\,(10^{5+6}) = 6 \times 10^{11}$$

The same method may be used for more complex numbers and calculations.

Example

$$2,230,000 \times 56,700 = 2.23 \times 10^6 \times 5.67 \times 10^4$$

or

$$2.23 \times 5.67\,(10^{6+4}) = 12.64 \times 10^{10} \text{ or } 1.264 \times 10^{11}$$

To multiply numbers expressed as negative powers of ten, first multiply the numbers (between 1 and 10) that are on the left of 10 to the minus power, then add the negative powers of ten.

$$0.000002 \times 0.0000003 = 2 \times 10^{-6} \times 3 \times 10^{-7} = 2 \times 3\,(10^{(-6)+(-7)}) = 6 \times 10^{-13}$$

The same scheme is followed to divide numbers expressed as powers of ten or negative powers of ten.

Example

$$\frac{600,000}{2000} = \frac{6 \times 10^5}{2 \times 10^3} = \frac{6\,(10^{5-3})}{2} = 3 \times 10^2 = 300$$

As seen in the above example, first divide the numbers (between 1 and 10) that are on the left of the powers or negative powers of ten, then subtract the power of ten in the denominator from that in the numerator. The following is an example of division of numbers expressed as negative powers of ten.

Example

$$\frac{0.0008}{0.00002} = \frac{8 \times 10^{-4}}{2 \times 10^{-5}} = \frac{8}{2}(10^{(-4)-(-5)}) = 4 \times 10^1 = 40$$

1.2 HANDLING FRACTIONS

A **simple fraction** is expressed as a ratio of two numbers (a numerator above the line and a denominator below) as, for example, $\frac{2}{3}, \frac{3}{4}$, or $\frac{1}{2}$. If the numerator is less than the denominator, as in the examples, the fraction is called a **proper fraction**. **Improper fractions** have larger numerators than denominators, as $\frac{5}{7}$ or $\frac{7}{4}$. Fractions may be added, subtracted, multiplied, or divided by following a few simple rules. To add or subtract fractions the quantities involved must be reduced to a **common denominator**.

Examples

In the addition of $\frac{2}{3} + \frac{3}{4} + \frac{1}{2}$ the common denominator is 12 since 12 is divisible by 3, 4, and 2. Therefore,

$$\frac{2}{3} + \frac{3}{4} + \frac{1}{2} = \frac{8}{12} + \frac{9}{12} + \frac{6}{12} = \frac{23}{12} = 1\frac{11}{12}$$

In subtraction of $3\frac{2}{3} - 1\frac{3}{4} - \frac{1}{2}$; the common denominator is 12. Therefore,

$$3\frac{2}{3} - 1\frac{3}{4} - \frac{1}{2} = 3\frac{8}{12} - 1\frac{9}{12} - \frac{6}{12} = \frac{42}{12} - \frac{21}{12} - \frac{6}{12} = \frac{17}{12} = 1\frac{5}{12}$$

To multiply simple fractions, first multiply the numerators; then multiply the denominators and finally reduce the resulting fraction to its lowest terms.

Examples

$$\frac{2}{3} \times \frac{3}{4} \times \frac{1}{2} = \frac{6}{24} = \frac{1}{4}$$

$$1\frac{2}{3} \times 2\frac{3}{4} \times 1\frac{1}{2} = \frac{5}{3} \times \frac{11}{4} \times \frac{3}{2} = \frac{165}{24} = 6\frac{21}{24} = 6\frac{7}{8}$$

To divide one fraction by another, invert the divisor and multiply.

Examples

$$\frac{3}{4} \div \frac{1}{2} = \frac{3}{4} \times \frac{2}{1} = \frac{6}{4} = 1\frac{2}{4} = 1\frac{1}{2}$$

$$2\frac{2}{3} \div \frac{3}{4} = \frac{8}{3} \times \frac{4}{3} = \frac{24}{9} = 2\frac{6}{9} = 2\frac{2}{3}$$

EXERCISES

A. $1\frac{1}{3} + \frac{3}{4} =$

B. $4\frac{2}{3} - 1\frac{1}{2} =$

C. $3\frac{3}{4} \times 2\frac{1}{3} =$

D. $6\frac{1}{2} \div 2\frac{2}{3} =$

E. $1\frac{3}{4} \times 1\frac{2}{3} \times 2\frac{1}{2} =$

A **decimal fraction** is a proper fraction with a denominator expressed as a power of 10, as for example $\frac{5}{10}$, $\frac{3}{100}$, and $\frac{7}{1000}$. Using a decimal point, these fractions can be simplified to the decimal fractions 0.5, 0.03, and 0.007. To change a proper fraction to a decimal fraction, divide the numerator by the denominator as, for example, $\frac{3}{5} = 0.6$ and $\frac{1}{4} = 0.25$. When adding or subtracting decimal fractions, the decimal points must always be in a vertical column.

WILLIAM F. MAAG LIBRARY
YOUNGSTOWN STATE UNIVERSITY
381161

Examples

0.5 + 0.03 + 0.007	2.05 - 1.006

$$
\begin{array}{l}
0.5 \\
0.03 \\
\underline{0.007} \\
0.537
\end{array}
\qquad
\begin{array}{l}
2.050 \\
\underline{1.006} \\
1.044
\end{array}
$$

When multiplying decimal fractions, the product must contain as many decimal places as the sum of the places to the right of the decimal in the numbers multiplied.

Examples

$$2.5 \times 3.45 = 8.625$$

$$1.05 \times 6.75 = 7.0875$$

When dividing decimal fractions, the quotient must contain as many decimal places as there are places in the dividend minus the number of places in the divisor. If zeros are added to the dividend, they are counted as decimal places.

Examples

$$3.45 \div 2.5 \qquad\qquad 9.275 \div 3.5$$

$$
\begin{array}{r}
1.38 \\
2.5\overline{)3.450} \\
\underline{2.5} \\
95 \\
\underline{75} \\
200
\end{array}
\qquad\qquad
\begin{array}{r}
2.65 \\
3.5\overline{)9.275} \\
\underline{7.0} \\
227 \\
\underline{210} \\
175
\end{array}
$$

WILLIAM F. MANG LIB
YOUNGS

EXERCISES

F. $0.75 + 0.3 + 0.275 =$

G. $20.65 - 4.25 =$

H. $3.55 \times 6.35 =$

I. $8.375 \div 2.5 =$

Fractional exponents of numbers expressed as powers of ten are commonly written using the root sign, $\sqrt{}$. For example, $10,000^{1/2} = \sqrt{10,000} = \sqrt{10^4}$, and $1000^{1/3} = \sqrt[3]{1000} = \sqrt[3]{10^3}$. When expressed as a square root, $\sqrt{}$, of a power of ten the value is obtained by dividing the exponent by two.

Examples

$$\sqrt{10,000} = \sqrt{10^4} = 10^{4/2} = 10^2 = 100$$

$$\sqrt{400} = \sqrt{4 \times 100} = \sqrt{4 \times 10^2} = 2 \times 10 = 20$$

The cube root, $\sqrt[3]{}$, of a power of ten is obtained by dividing the exponent by three.

Examples

$$\sqrt[3]{1000} = \sqrt[3]{10^3} = 10^{3/3} = 10$$

$$\sqrt[3]{0.000008} = \sqrt[3]{8 \times 10^{-6}} = 2 \times 10^{-2}$$

It is obvious that all of the above examples have powers of ten readily divided by the root (either 2 or 3). Many other examples of fractional exponents of numbers require logarithms for accurate calculations, as will be outlined in the next chapter.

EXERCISES

J. $\sqrt{900}$ =

K. $\sqrt{0.0001}$ =

L. $\sqrt[3]{10^{-9}}$ =

M. $\sqrt[3]{8000000}$ =

1.3 ESTABLISHING THE ANSWER AND THE CORRECT DECIMAL POINT

A major problem in laboratory calculations is the proper setting of the decimal point in the final calculated value. An example of the change of volume of a gas with a change in pressure and temperature may lead to the following calculation:

$$V = 625 \times \frac{810 \times 283}{730 \times 353}$$

An inspection of the two fractions 810/730 and 283/353 reveals that they will about balance each other and yield a value close to 1 to be multiplied times 625, so the answer should approximate 625. Actually it is 555, but the decimal is correct and the answer makes sense. A calculation whose answer has a decimal point that may be more difficult to set would be as follows:

$$\frac{95.62 \times 1.211 \times 6.78 \times 3.45}{22.31 \times 3.1416 \times 9.965}$$

In this type of problem we simplify the approximate solution by rounding off values and judiciously give and take on the values. You might reason as follows:

$$\frac{100 \times 1 \times 10 \times 2}{20 \times 3 \times 10}$$

Mentally $100 \times 10 = 1000 \times 2 = 2000$ divided by $20 \times 3 = 60 \times 10 = 600$ and 2000/600 is the same as 20/6, or approximately 3.3; the correct answer is close to 3.88.

Other calculations may not result in such a simple setting of the decimal point in the answer. The knowledge gained in Section 1.1 may be used to establish the correct answer and decimal point in more complex calculations:

$$\frac{200,000 \times 3000 \times 0.0004}{500 \times 0.0012 \times 10,000} = \frac{2 \times 10^5 \times 3 \times 10^3 \times 4 \times 10^{-4}}{5 \times 10^2 \times 1.2 \times 10^{-3} \times 1 \times 10^4}$$

Since to multiply we add the powers of ten, the fraction would be expressed as:

$$\frac{2 \times 3 \times 4}{5 \times 1.2 \times 1} \times \frac{10^{5+3+(-4)}}{10^{2+(-3)+4}} = 4 \times \frac{10^4}{10^3}$$

To divide we subtract the power of ten in the denominator from that in the numerator, or $4 \times 10^{4-3} = 4 \times 10 = 40$. Manipulation of a series of more complex numbers may be illustrated as follows:

$$\frac{1232 \times 3.141 \times 627.6 \times 72.1}{29.42 \times 411.2 \times 6.95}$$

As powers of ten:

$$\frac{1.232 \times 10^3 \times 3.141 \times 6.276 \times 10^2 \times 7.21 \times 10^1}{2.942 \times 10^1 \times 4.112 \times 10^2 \times 6.95}$$

$$= \frac{1.232 \times 3.141 \times 6.276 \times 7.21}{2.942 \times 4.112 \times 6.95} \times \frac{10^{3+2}}{10^2}$$

$$= \text{approx.} \ \frac{1 \times 3 \times 6 \times 7}{3 \times 4 \times 7} = \frac{126}{84} \times 10^{5-2} = 1.8 \times 10^3$$

$$= \text{by actual calculation } 2.08 \times 10^3 = 2080$$

In laboratory calculations it is often of great assistance to know the range of values expected from a patient and thus from the method and the proper calculation of values by the use of that method. There are many instances in which the method and the calculation are properly designed to yield, for example, values in a range of 5 to 20 mg/dl. It is always somewhat of a shock when a laboratory technician insists that the patient's blood level is 143 mg/dl because he obtained that answer from his calculation. The use of common sense in this calculation implies not only knowing how to establish the correct decimal point but also recognizing the range of levels you would ordinarily expect. Before insisting on 143 mg/dl or even entering it in the patient's record, it would be wise to recalculate the problem.

ADDITIONAL EXERCISES

1. If peaches were priced at $0.77 a kilogram, what would they cost per pound?

2. Some professional football players can command an annual salary equivalent to their weight in gold. If gold sells for $1000 a kilogram and a player weighs 220 pounds, what is his annual salary?

3. A technician's child appeared to be running a high fever. The only thermometer available was calibrated in degrees centigrade and gave a reading of 40°C. What was the child's temperature in degrees Fahrenheit?

4. Dry ice and acetone mixtures are often used for the rapid freezing of biological specimens. A temperature of –80°C may be obtained in this fashion. Express this in degrees Fahrenheit.

5. Room temperature is usually about 70°F. What would be the reading on the centigrade scale?

6. In the following examples give the approximate answer obtained by mental arithmetic to aid in setting the correct decimal point.

    a. $\dfrac{1152.6 \times 3.1416 \times 809.61}{38.46 \times 12.124 \times 4.891}$

    b. $633 \times \dfrac{820}{760} \times \dfrac{290}{353}$

    c. $\dfrac{24.782 \times 2.173 \times 111.22}{42.36 \times 9.77 \times 2.676}$

7. Express the following numbers as powers of ten or negative powers of ten.

    a. 2,200,000   d. 0.0003

    b. 46,000   e. 0.00000044

    c. 151,000   f. 0.000000005

8. Carry out the following calculations after first converting to powers or negative powers of ten.

    a. 410000 × 23000

    b. 5600000 × 720000

    c. 0.000031 × 0.00022

    d. $\dfrac{8100000}{300000}$

2
Logarithms

THE *PRACTICAL OBJECTIVES* OF THIS CHAPTER ARE TO OBTAIN AN UNDERSTANDING OF:

1. The basis of logarithms, the characteristic and mantissa.

2. The use of logarithm tables to find logarithms and antilogarithms.

3. The use of logarithms in multiplication, division, powers and roots of numbers.

The logarithm of a number is the power to which a given base must be raised to equal that number. In the common system of logarithms the base is always 10. For example, $1000 = 10^3$, so the logarithm of 1000 to the base 10 is 3. Similarly 2 is the logarithm of 100 because $10^2 = 100$. Also 0.699 is the logarithm of 5 since $10^{0.699} = 5$. In the preceding chapter we have seen that small fractions or numbers less than one (1.0) can be expressed as 10 to a minus power. For example, $0.001 = 10^{-3}$ and the logarithm of 0.001 would be -3. The figure 0.1 can be expressed as 10^{-1} and thus has a logarithm of -1. It should not be too difficult to decide that the log of $1 = 0$ and that the log of $10 = 1$. Most logarithms are not as simple as the above examples and consist of two major parts, the **characteristic** and **mantissa**. The logarithm of 752, for example, is 2.8762; in this example the number to the left of the decimal point, 2, is called the characteristic, and the decimal part, 0.8762, is called the mantissa.

2.1 THE CHARACTERISTIC

The characteristic of the logarithm of a number equal to or greater than one is one less than the number of digits to the left of the decimal point. The characteristic of the log of 752 would then be 2, while that of 75.2 would be 1 and the characteristic of 7.52 would be 0.

Examples

The characteristic of 6271 $= 3$

$$1.5 = 0$$
$$30.2 = 1$$
$$512 = 2$$

The characteristic of the logarithm of a number less than one is negative and is one more than the number of zeros after the decimal point. A negative characteristic may be expressed by placing a negative sign over the number, as $\bar{1}$, $\bar{2}$ or $\bar{3}$, or as a positive number minus 10; that is $\bar{1}$ would be 9 – 10, $\bar{2}$ would be 8 – 10 and $\bar{3}$ would be expressed as 7 – 10. The use of a negative characteristic with a positive mantissa in the log of 0.005 = $\bar{3}$, or the subtraction of the 3 from 10 – 10 to give 7 – 10, is employed in most calculations involving logarithms.

Examples

The characteristic of 0.005 = $\bar{3}$ or 7 – 10
0.10 = $\bar{1}$ or 9 – 10
0.025 = $\bar{2}$ or 8 – 10

2.2 THE MANTISSA

The mantissa is the decimal part of the logarithm and is independent of the decimal point in the original number. The mantissa of the log of a number is found in logarithm tables, and although the decimal points are not printed in the table, each mantissa is understood to have a decimal point in front of it. The L scale of a slide rule may also be used to obtain the mantissa. This procedure will be explained in the following section. The logarithm table (see the Appendix at the end of this book) contains mantissas of numbers from 1 to 9999 to four decimal places. This is called a four-place table and has the first two digits of the number in the left column under N with the third in a row across the top from 0 to 9. All of the numbers in the body of the table from 0000 to 9996 are mantissas. The mantissa of a two digit number is found under the 0 column opposite the number; for example, the mantissa of 65 is 0.8129. For a three digit number the mantissa is found under the column corresponding to the third digit opposite the first two digits; thus the mantissa of 455 is 0.6580.

Examples

The mantissa of   5.0 = 0.6990
56 = 0.7482
820 = 0.9138
82 = 0.9138
8.2 = 0.9138

2.3 THE LOGARITHM OF A NUMBER

To find the complete logarithm of a number we first establish the characteristic and follow it with the mantissa as the decimal part found in logarithm tables. A four-place table yields mantissas of three digit numbers directly and four digit numbers by interpolation between the numbers across the top of the table. The use of the four-place table will be illustrated in the following examples.

Example

Find the log of 672. The characteristic is 2, and the mantissa from the tables is 0.8274, so the complete logarithm of 672 is 2.8274. Finding the log of 6725 involves an additional step. The characteristic is 3, and the mantissa is determined as follows:

$$\text{The mantissa of } 6720 = 0.8274$$
$$6730 = 0.8280$$
$$6725 = 0.8277$$

$$
\begin{array}{r}
0.8280 \\
-0.8274 \\
\hline
0.0006 \\
0.5 \\
\hline
0.0003
\end{array}
$$

The reasoning would be as follows. 6725 is half of the way (0.5) between 6720 and 6730, whose mantissas are 0.8274 and 0.8280, respectively, with a difference of 0.0006; 0.5 of 0.0006 is 0.0003. Adding this to 0.8274 = 0.8277, the mantissa of 6725. The complete logarithm would then be 3.8277. You will notice that the logarithm table has a set of proportional parts to assist you in interpolation between the last two digits. In any horizontal row in the table the difference between the 10 mantissas is nearly the same number, and the number across the top of the proportional parts set are tenths of the difference between any two mantissas in that row. A satisfactory logarithm of 6725 could be obtained by following the characteristic of 3 with the mantissa obtained by reading the 672 from the table as 0.8274 and adding the proportional part in that row under the 5 on the top, giving 0.0003 + 0.8274 = 0.8277, or a log of 3.8277. A few practice examples will establish this principle in your mind.

EXERCISES

Find the logarithm of

A. 5.5   =   _____

B. 431   =   _____

C. 0.062 =   _____

D. 3244 =   _____

E. 0.15 =   _____

2.4 THE NUMBER CORRESPONDING TO A GIVEN LOGARITHM

To find the number that corresponds to a particular logarithm we have to reverse the process of finding the logarithm. This may be done with a slide rule (as will be explained later), by use of a table of **antilogarithms** (see Appendix; reverse logarithms may be a better name) or by finding the digits in the number that correspond to the mantissa of the logarithm in a regular log table and setting the decimal point from the characteristics of the logarithm. As an example let us find the number whose logarithm is 2.4843. The mantissa 0.4843 is located in the row whose first two digits are 30 and is under the third digit 5 in the top row. The three digits are therefore 305 and with a characteristic of 2 would have three digits to the left of the decimal point, resulting in the number 305. We can then say the log of 305 is 2.4843, or the reverse logarithm, or antilogarithm, of 2.4843 is 3.05×10^2, or 305. The same example can be solved directly by use of the table of antilogarithms. In this table the first two digits of the mantissa are given as decimals in the left column, while the third digit is shown across the top and the fourth digit of the mantissa is found by use of the proportional parts. The number corresponding to the logarithm is given in the body of the table from 1000 to 9977. To obtain the digits of the number from the mantissa 0.4843 we start with the row having 0.48 on the left side then move over to the number 3048 under the 4 column and add 2 as the proportional part under 3, giving the four digits 3050. Again, with a characteristic of 2 the number corresponding to a log of 2.4843 would be 3.05×10^2, or 305.

When dealing with logarithms with negative characteristics, we must first rewrite the log in the form of a decimal fraction between 0 and 1.0000 minus a whole number. For example, to find the number whose log is $\bar{3}.6195$ or $7.6195 - 10$, we write it as $0.6195 - 3$ and determine the antilog of the mantissa, 0.6195 × antilog – 3. From the table of antilogarithms, 0.6195 corresponds to 4.164, and since the antilog of – 3 is 10^{-3}, the number is 4.164 × 10^{-3}, or 0.004164.

Examples

Find the number that corresponds to log 4.3784.

antilog of mantissa 0.3784 = 2.390, so antilog of 4.3784 = 2.390 × antilog 4 = 2.390 × 10^4 = 23,900;

or

log 4.3784 = 0.3784 + 4;

number = antilog 0.3784 × antilog +4 = 2.390 × 10^4 = 23,900.

log $\overline{5}$.1802 = 5.1802 – 10 = 0.1802 – 5

number = antilog 0.1802 × antilog –5 = 1.515 × 10^{-5} = 0.00001515

EXERCISES

Find the antilog of

A.   1.3177 = _____

B.   3.1805 = _____

C.   0.2664 = _____

D. $\overline{2}$.5768 or 8.5768 – 10 = _____

E. $\overline{1}$.3667 or 9.3667 – 10 = _____

2.5 MULTIPLICATION

Calculations with the aid of logarithms follow the laws of exponents, since logarithms are actually exponents. **The logarithm of the product of two numbers is the sum of their logarithms.**

$$\log ab = \log a + \log b$$

To multiply numbers, add their logarithms and find the number that corresponds to that logarithm (the antilogarithm).

Examples

$$12.6 \times 4.3 = 54.18$$

$$
\begin{aligned}
\log \ 12.6 &= 1.1004 \\
\log \ \ 4.3 &= \underline{0.6335} \\
\text{sum} \ \ \ &= 1.7339
\end{aligned}
$$

antilog of $1.7339 = 5.418 \times 10^1 = 54.18$

$$3.2 \times 0.063 \times 15.6 = 3.145$$

$$
\begin{aligned}
\log \ \ 3.2 \ \ &= \ \ 0.5051 \\
\log \ \ 0.063 \ &= \ \ 8.7993 - 10 \\
\log 15.6 \ \ &= \ \ \underline{1.1931} \\
\text{sum} \ \ \ \ \ \ &= 10.4975 - 10 \text{ or } 0.4975
\end{aligned}
$$

antilog of $0.4975 = 3.145$

EXERCISES

A. 1.35×14.6 = _____

B. $32.6 \times 0.57 \times 17.1$ = _____

C. $0.004 \times 0.128 \times 6.3$ = _____

2.6 DIVISION

From the properties of exponents, **the logarithm of the quotient of two numbers is equal to the logarithm of the numerator minus the logarithm of the denominator.**

$$\log \frac{a}{b} = \log a - \log b$$

To divide numbers, subtract the logarithm of the denominator from the logarithm of the numerator and find the number that corresponds to that logarithm (antilogarithm).

Examples

$$\frac{205.1}{62.6} = 3.27$$

log 205.1 = 2.3120
log 62.6 = 1.7966
difference = 0.5154
antilog of 0.5154 = 3.276

Another example combining multiplication and division

$$\frac{35.6 \times 0.72 \times 14.9}{11.3 \times 0.082} = 412.1$$

log 35.6   =   1.5514
log   0.72 =   9.8573 – 10
log 14.9   =   1.1732
sum   = 12.5819 – 10

log 11.3   =   1.0531
log 0.082 =   8.9138 – 10
sum   =   9.9669 – 10

to divide: 12.5819 – 10
          9.9669 – 10
          2.6150
antilog of 2.6150 = 4.121 $\times 10^2$ = 412.1

EXERCISES

A. $\dfrac{4.15}{0.86}$ = _____

B. $\dfrac{15.2 \times 12.6}{5.76}$ = _____

C. $\dfrac{21.1 \times 4.3 \times 622.2}{3.76 \times 29.8} =$ _____

2.7 POWERS OF NUMBERS

The logarithm of a number to the nth power is n times the logarithm of the number.

$$\log a^n = n \log a$$

To raise a number to a power, multiply the logarithm of the number by the power and find the number that corresponds to the logarithm (antilogarithm).

Examples

To evaluate 4.5^3

$$
\begin{array}{lll}
\log (4.5)^3 & = & 3 \times \log 4.5 \\
\log 4.5 & = & 0.6532 \\
& & \underline{\times\ 3} \\
& & 1.9596
\end{array}
$$

antilog of $1.9596 = 9.110 \times 10^1 = 91.10$

To calculate 14.23^2

$$
\begin{array}{lll}
\log (14.23)^2 & = & 2 \times \log 14.23 \\
\log 14.23 & = & 1.1532 \\
& & \underline{\times\ 2} \\
& & 2.3064
\end{array}
$$

antilog of $2.3064 = 2.025 \times 10^2 = 202.5$

2.8 ROOTS

The logarithm of a number to the nth root is the logarithm of the number divided by n.

$$\log \sqrt[n]{a} = \frac{1}{n} \log a = \frac{\log a}{n}$$

To determine the nth root of a number, divide the logarithm of the number by the root and find the number that corresponds to the divided logarithm (antilogarithm).

Examples

To find $\sqrt[3]{32.2}$

$$\log \sqrt[3]{32.2} = \frac{1}{3} \log 32.2$$

$$\log 32.2 = \frac{1.5079}{3} = 0.5026$$

antilog of 0.5026 = 3.181

To determine $\sqrt{1026}$

$$\log \sqrt{1026} = \frac{1}{2} \log 1026$$

$$\log 1026 = \frac{3.0111}{2} = 1.5055$$

antilog of 1.5055 = 3.203×10^1 = 32.03

2.9 LOGARITHM OF NUMBERS EXPRESSED AS POWERS OF TEN

In chemical calculations, concentrations are often expressed as powers of ten. For example, we may use 5.6×10^8 moles of a substance or a hydrogen ion concentration of 2.5×10^{-4}. The general expression would be $a \times 10^b$ where the logarithm equals:

$$\log a + \log 10^b = b + \log a$$

Examples

$$\log 5.6 \times 10^8 = \log 5.6 + \log 10^8 = 8 + \log 5.6$$

$$\log 5.6 = 0.7482 \text{ and } 8 + 0.7482 = 8.7482$$
$$\text{Therefore } \log 5.6 \times 10^8 = 8.7482$$

$$\text{To check antilog} = 560,000,000 \text{ or } 5.6 \times 10^8$$

$$\log 2.5 \times 10^{-4} = \log 2.5 + \log 10^{-4} = -4 + \log 2.5$$

$$\log 2.5 = 0.3979 \text{ and } -4 + 0.3979 = \overline{4}.3979 = 6.3979 - 10$$

$$\text{To check antilog} = 0.00025 = 2.5 \times 10^{-4}$$

EXERCISES

A. 776^2 = _____

B. 35.1^3 = _____

C. $\sqrt{86.2}$ = _____

D. $\log 7.2 \times 10^6$ = _____

E. $\log 5.2 \times 10^{-3}$ = _____

ADDITIONAL EXERCISES

1. Give the characteristic of the logarithm of the following:

a. 423

b. 0.032

c. 0.00005

   d. 23.5

   e. 1.7

2. Give the mantissa of the logarithm of the following:

   a. 4.6

   b. 460

   c. 78

   d. 0.143

   e. 0.007

3. What is the logarithm of the following numbers?

   a. 672

   b. 1.5

   c. 34000

   d. 0.0034

4. What is the antilogarithm of the following logarithms?

   a. 2.7810

   b. 0.5988

   c. 8.4440 – 10

   d. 1.9877

   e. 7.6314 – 10

5. Carry out the following calculations using logarithms.

   a. 35 × 66

   b. 1.68 × 5600

   c. $3.1416 \times 620 \times 15$

   d. $\dfrac{3200}{27}$

   e. $\dfrac{0.002 \times 28.5 \times 143.5}{2.47 \times 3.1416}$

6. Work the following problems with logarithms.

   a. 17.56^3

   b. 1.46^2

   c. $\sqrt[3]{42.3}$

   d. $\log 8.1 \times 10^5$

   e. $\log 2.4 \times 10^{-6}$

3

The Slide Rule

THE *PRACTICAL OBJECTIVES* OF THE CHAPTER ARE TO OBTAIN AN UNDERSTANDING OF:

1. The scales and settings of the slide rule.

2. The use of the slide rule in rapid solution of problems involving multiplication, division, squares, and square roots.

3. The advantages of the circular slide rule and its use in calculations.

A slide rule is a simple instrument containing several scales on which **whole numbers are spaced at intervals proportional to their logarithms.** This arrangement permits rapid mechanical calculations by the use of logarithms and antilogarithms. **Multiplications,** for example, are carried out by **adding logarithms** of numbers and reading the antilogarithm of the answer. **Divisions** are readily carried out by the opposite manipulation of **subtracting logarithms** and reading the antilogarithm of the answer on a slide rule scale.

A careful examination of an inexpensive slide rule will reveal three major parts, the body, the slide and the indicator with a hairline. The **body** usually has scales such as the A, D, K, and L scales. The **slide** has projections on the sides that are closely fitted into grooves on the body of the slide rule for smooth back-and-forth movement. The slide ordinarily has B, C and C_1 scales plus special scales for various calculations. The **indicator** consists of a window with a vertical hairline; the indicator slides smoothly in grooves on the outer edges of the body of the slide rule.

A comparison of the C and D scales with the L scale will reveal the basis for multiplication and division by use of logarithms on the slide rule. The L scale is linear with equal spaces between the 10 major numbers; these divisions correspond to the mantissa of logarithms found in a log table. The C and D scales also contain 10 major divisions, but the whole numbers are spaced at distances proportional to their logarithms. For example, the log of 2 is 0.301, so the 2 is located over the 0.301 on the linear or log scale L. In like manner the log of 5 is 0.699, so the 5 is located over the 0.699 on the L scale. Also, since the log of 10 is 1.000, the number 10 on the extreme right of the C or D scales is over the 1.000 on the L scale.

FIGURE 3.1

3.1 THE DIVISION OF NUMBERS ON THE SLIDE RULE

A major problem for students first learning to use a slide rule is the division of whole numbers on the C and D scales. To correctly read the scales on a slide rule you must be thoroughly familiar with the major and minor divisions of each whole number. If we first consider the whole number divisions on the C and D scales, they will appear as in Figure 3.2.

FIGURE 3.2

The space between each whole number is first divided into tenths, making it relatively simple to read the first two digits of a given number. Further division of the tenths between each whole number varies with the size of the space between the numbers, as seen in Figure 3.3. The large space between 1 and 2 permits each tenth to be divided into tenths, for a total of 100 divisions, allowing a direct reading of the first three digits with the fourth digit to be estimated. An example of a number setting in this region would be 166 or 1660; move the hairline of the indicator to the right of the 1 on the D scale to the 6 (6 tenths mark) and then to the 6th mark between 6 and 7 (6 hundredth mark). This setting of 166 could represent 1660, 0.166, 16.6 or any other combination of 166. If the value was 1665, you would further move the hairline to the right halfway between the 6th and 7th hundredth mark.

FIGURE 3.3

The area between whole numbers 2 and 4 is first divided into tenths (these divisions are not marked with numbers as they are between 1 and 2). The smaller space permits only further divisions of fifths between the tenths making a total of 50 divisions between 2 and 3 and between 3 and 4. The smallest divisions would thus represent 2 hundredths instead of 1 hundredth as between 1 and 2. A setting of 366 would be achieved by moving the hairline past 3 to the right to the 6 tenth mark and then to the third division (6 hundredths) between the 6th and 7th tenth. To set 367 you would further move the hairline halfway between third and fourth division (6th and 8th hundredths) between the 6th and 7th tenth.

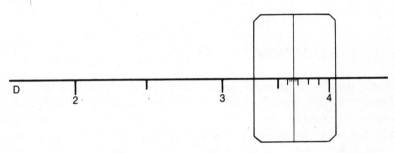

FIGURE 3.4

For whole numbers 4 to 10 each number is again divided into tenths, and each tenth is divided into halves, making the smallest divisions 5 hundredths. There would thus be 20 divisions between each whole number from 4 to 10. To set the number 665 you would move the hairline past 6 to the right to the 6th tenth and then to the mark halfway between the 6th and 7th tenth. In this region of the D scale the third digit of a number must be estimated by the spacing between the tenths if it is any number other than 5.

FIGURE 3.5

Before attempting any calculations with the slide rule, practice setting numbers on the D scale with the hairline. For example, locate the following numbers and check your setting with the log values from the L scale.

Examples

Set 126   (corresponds to 0.100 on L scale)
    3.16 (corresponds to 0.500 on L scale)
  1675   (corresponds to 0.224 on L scale)
    45.5 (corresponds to 0.658 on L scale)
   867   (corresponds to 0.938 on L scale)
    6.31 (corresponds to 0.800 on L scale)
  1333   (corresponds to 0.125 on L scale)

3.2 MULTIPLICATION

Since the C and D scale numbers correspond to the mantissa of the logarithms on the L scale, the process of multiplication on the slide rule consists of adding the logarithm of two numbers and finding the number corresponding to the sum of the logarithms on the D scale. A simple example would be to multiply 2 × 2. First set the 1 on the left of the C scale over the 2 on the D scale; then move the hairline to the 2 on the C scale and read the answer below on the D scale. The answer is obviously 4, but this is also an easy one to understand – addition of the log of 2 = 0.301 (from 0 to 0.301 on the L scale) and the log of 2, or

$$0.301 + 0.301 = 0.602$$

on the L scale, which corresponds to the number or antilog of 4.

FIGURE 3.6

In general you use the 1 on the C scale at either the left or right end of the slide rule, depending on the number you are multiplying. For example, you wish to multiply 4 × 5. You will find that if you set the 1 on the left of the C scale over the 4 on the D scale, the 5 on the C scale projects out into space. By setting the

1 on the right side of the C scale over the 4 on the D scale, the hairline can be moved to the 5 on the C scale and the answer 20 found below the line on the D scale. To try a more difficult example multiply 185 X 4.46. Set the 1 on the left of the C scale over 185 and move the hairline to 4, then to 4 tenths and then to 6 hundredths, or 446, and find the answer 825 below on the D scale. Practice multiplication by working the following problems.

EXERCISES

A. 15 X 39   = _____

B. 21 X 35   = _____

C. 92 X 6.85 = _____

D. 52 X 2.5 = _____

3.3 SETTING THE DECIMAL POINT

In both multiplication and division problems on the slide rule there is a rather complex method of setting the decimal point of an answer that involves the span of a number, the sum or difference between spans and the addition or subtraction of 1 from the sum or difference of the spans, depending on which side of the slide rule the C slide projects. Unfortunately a wrong answer could result from the improper use of the span method even after the correct slide rule manipulation was carried out. **The common sense approach explained in Section 1.3** will assist you in setting the correct decimal point in your answer. The procedure of multiplying two numbers such as 1.95 X 33.6 would begin with setting the 1 on the left of the C scale over the 195 on the D scale and moving the hairline to the 336 on the C scale; the answer is 656. The problem is the decimal point; should the correct answer be 6.56, 65.6, 656? By rounding off the figures 1.95 to 2 and 33.6 to 30 the answer would be approximately 60; 65.6 is therefore correct. In every problem in which the answer is not readily apparent the decimal point setting should be determined by rounding off the numbers and obtaining an approximate answer. As stated earlier, this process can usually be worked out mentally and is worthy of practice.

3.4 MULTIPLICATION OF MORE THAN TWO NUMBERS

Laboratory calculations often involve the multiplication of three or more factors, a process which can readily be carried out on the slide rule. Take as an example the problem 3.14 × 52.6 × 0.935. First, set the 1 on the right of the C scale over 3.14 on the D scale, then move the hairline to 52.6 on the C scale. Instead of reading the answer as 165.1 on the D scale move the 1 on the right of the C scale to the hairline setting (165.1) and then move the hairline to 935 on the C scale and read the answer 1528 below on the D scale. You should be able to set the decimal by inspection since 0.935 is almost 1 and 3 × 50 equals 150 so the correct answer would be 152.8. With the hairline on the setting 1528 on the D scale you could complete the four number problem 3.14 × 52.6 × 0.935 × 75 by moving the 1 on the right of the C scale to the hairline setting (1528) and again moving the hairline to the 75 on the C scale reading the answer 1147 below on the C scale. To set the decimal point multiply 150 × 70 mentally, obtaining 10500; so the correct answer would be 11,470. Do the following exercises to gain proficiency in multiplication and the setting of the decimal point.

EXERCISES

		Approximate answer
A.	5.2 × 0.876 × 12.3	= 5 × 1 × 10 = 50
B.	94.3 × 18.1 × 31.2	= 100 × 20 × 30 = 60,000
C.	7.8 × 5.6 × 19.2 × 62.3 =	10 × 5 × 20 × 60 = 60,000
D.	46.4 × 0.082 × 3.33	= 50 × 0.1 × 3 = 15
E.	110.5 × 2.56 × 0.0094	= 100 × 3 × 0.01 = 3

3.5 DIVISION

Division on the slide rule involves a logarithmic process by which the logarithm of the denominator is subtracted from the logarithm of the numerator, and the number corresponding to the differences between the logarithms is found on the D scale. Employing the example, 4/2, or 4 divided by 2, we set the denominator 2 on the C scale directly over the numerator 4 on the D scale and moving the hairline to the 1 on the C scale find the answer 2 below on the D scale. This is the exact reverse of multiplication (2 × 2 = 4). Also in division we subtract the log of 2 = 0.301 from the log of 4 = 0.602 to obtain the log

$$0.602 - 0.301 = 0.301$$

which corresponds to the number 2, which is the answer.

FIGURE 3.7

Another example will illustrate that the manipulation for division is the reverse of that for multiplication. In the problem 30/2 = 15 we also see that 15 X 2 = 30. On the slide rule to divide 30/2 we would set 2 on the C scale over 30 on the D scale and read 15 on the D scale under the 1 on the C scale, or to reverse the process and multiply 15 x 2, we would set the 1 on the C scale over 15 and move the hairline to 2 on the C scale to find the answer 30 below on the D scale.

Example

Approximate answer	Correct answer
$\dfrac{52.5}{2.5} = \dfrac{50}{2} = 25$	21.0

Note: The hairline should be used to line up properly the 52.5 on the D scale with the 2.5 on the C scale.

EXERCISES

Approximate answer

A. $\dfrac{111.1}{12.6} = \dfrac{100}{10} = 10$

B. $\dfrac{5280}{2.25}$ = $\dfrac{5000}{2}$ = 2500

C. $\dfrac{1.875}{0.0085}$ = $\dfrac{2}{0.01}$ = 200

3.6 COMBINATION MULTIPLICATION AND DIVISION PROBLEMS

Frequently a calculation in the laboratory will involve both multiplication and division. These problems can be rapidly solved by the use of the slide rule. An example might be $\dfrac{4 \times 30}{6}$ where you could first carry out the multiplication and then divide the answer by 6 as follows: Set the 1 on the right of the C scale over 4 on the D scale; then move the hairline to the 3 on the C scale and find 120 below on the D scale. Now move the 6 on the C scale to the hairline over the 120 on the D scale, and the answer 20 is found on the D scale under the 1 on the right side of the C scale. To carry the process further, divide 4 × 30 × 8 by 6 × 3, or solve the problem $\dfrac{4 \times 30 \times 8}{6 \times 3}$. First multiply all the numbers by setting the 1 on the right side of the C scale over 8 on the D scale, then move the hairline to 4 on the C scale, which is over 32 on the D scale; next move the 1 on the left of the C scale over the hairline (32) and move the hairline to 3 on the C scale, which is over 960 on the D scale. Then to divide move the 6 on the C scale over the hairline (960) on the D scale and find 160 on the D scale under the 1 on the left of the C scale; finally move the 3 on the C scale over the hairline at 160 on the D scale, and by moving to the 1 on the right of the C scale you will find the answer 53.3 on the D scale.

Since so many problems will involve calculations such as $\dfrac{5 \times 22 \times 7}{3 \times 4}$, we will illustrate another slide rule method that may involve fewer manipulations; you may choose the method most easy to remember and to carry out for a particular problem. In this method you first divide and then multiply and alternate these operations until the problem is complete. First divide 5 by 3 by setting 3 on the C scale over 5 on the D scale; then multiply the answer on the D scale (167) by 22 merely by moving the hairline to 22 on the C scale, since the 1 on the C scale is already over the 167. Then divide the answer 367 on the D scale by 4 by setting 4 on the C scale over the hairline on 367 on the D scale; finally multiply the value 917 on the D scale by 7 by moving the hairline to 7 on the C scale, since again the 1 on the right side of the C scale is already set over the 917 on the D scale. The complete answer is found under the 7 on the C scale and is 641 on the D scale. The approximate answer is

$$\frac{5 \times 20 \times 7}{12} = \frac{700}{12} = 60$$

so the correct decimal setting is 64.1. With practice the method just described will save considerable time in a series of calculations.

Since these combination problems are commonly encountered in laboratory methods, we will work our way through another example before the practice problems. An extra long example would be:

$$\frac{4.25 \times 6.1 \times 23.3 \times 19.6}{0.38 \times 11.1 \times 8.9}$$

which we will work by **the alternate division-multiplication method**. First, divide 4.25 by 0.38 by setting 38 on the C scale over 425 on the D scale; then multiply the answer 1119 by 6.1 by moving the hairline to 61, since the 1 on the C scale is already set over 1119. Next divide the answer 682 by 11.1 by setting 11.1 on the C scale over the 682 under the hairline on the D scale; then multiply the answer 614 by 23.3 by setting the 1 on the right side of the C scale over 614 and moving the hairline to the 23.3 on the C scale. The answer 143 is next divided by 8.9 by moving the 8.9 on the C scale over the hairline at 143; the answer 1609 is finally multiplied by 19.6 by moving the 1 (on the left of the C scale) over the 1609 and moving the hairline to the 19.6 on the C scale to give the final answer 315. The approximate answer is $\frac{4 \times 6 \times 20 \times 20}{0.4 \times 10 \times 10} = 240$, so the correct decimal setting is 315.

EXERCISES

Approximate answer

A. $\dfrac{35 \times 3}{9}$ $= \dfrac{30 \times 3}{10} = 9$

B. $\dfrac{5 \times 12.5 \times 55}{4 \times 11}$ $= \dfrac{5 \times 10 \times 60}{5 \times 10} = 60$

C. $\dfrac{3.14 \times 67.2}{5.25 \times 8.95}$ $= \dfrac{3 \times 70}{5 \times 10} = 4.2$

D. $\dfrac{510 \times 6.1 \times 21.3}{4.98 \times 0.071} = \dfrac{500 \times 6 \times 20}{5 \times 0.01} = 120{,}000$

E. $\dfrac{17.2 \times 22.2 \times 9.3}{898 \times 0.212} = \dfrac{20 \times 20 \times 10}{1000 \times 0.2} = 20$

3.7 SQUARES AND SQUARE ROOTS

Both the **squares** and **square roots** of numbers are commonly encountered in quality control work in the laboratory. The manipulations to solve this type of problem on the slide rule **involve only the D and A scales** without the use of the sliding C scale.

To find the square of a number set the hairline over that number on the D scale and read the answer on the A scale under the hairline. You will observe that the A scale is a double scale, containing the numbers on the C or D scale on each half. The squaring of simple numbers such as 2 and 4 will illustrate the utility of the double scale. Set the hairline over the 2 on the D scale and read 4 under the hairline on the A scale ($2^2 = 4$). Also set the hairline over the 4 on the D scale and read 16 under the hairline on the A scale ($4^2 = 16$). To square 29.2 set the hairline on 292 on the D scale and read 852 on the A scale. To set the decimal point round off 29.2 to 30, square it mentally and obtain 900. The answer therefore, is 852.

Examples

Square the following numbers

Approximate answer

A. 3.67 $=$ $3 \times 3 = 9$

B. 22.2 $=$ $20 \times 20 = 400$

C. 6.98 $=$ $7 \times 7 = 49$

D. 816 $=$ $800 \times 800 = 640{,}000$

To find the square root of a number set the hairline over that number on the A scale and read the answer under the hairline on the D scale. Even though square roots are found by a method opposite to that used for finding the square of a number, the double A scale poses some problems. To decide which half of the A scale to use the simple scheme outlined below may be followed.

1. If the number is 1 or greater, space off groups of two digits from the decimal point to your **left**. If the last group to the left has one digit, use the left half of A; if the last group to the left has two digits, use the right half of A. For example, to find the square root of 676.0 divide the number two digits to the left of the decimal point (6/76); you will find one digit in the last group to the left. Setting 676 on the left half of A, the answer is 26. It is obvious that $26^2 = 676$ so the answer is correctly set at 26. In a quality control problem the sum of the squares may be 1459.0. To find the square root of 1459.0 first divide the digits to the left of the decimal point in groups of two (14/59). Since the last group to the left has two digits use the right side of the A scale. Setting 1459 on the right side of the A scale the answer under the hairline on the D scale is 382. To decide on the decimal point round off 382 to 400 and try 400 $\times$ 400 = 16,000, which is incorrect; so try 40 $\times$ 40 = 1600, which sets the correct number as 38.2.

2. If the number is less than 1, space off groups of two digits from the decimal point to your **right**. If the first group with a significant figure to right of the decimal point contains one number, use the left half of the A scale. If the first group contains two numbers, use the right half of the scale. To find the square root, for example, of 0.0096 again space off in groups of two (0.00/96). Since there are two numbers in the group with significant figures, we use the right half of scale A, setting 96 and reading 98 on the D scale.

It is more difficult to set the decimal point in square roots of numbers less than one so an arbitrary scheme is used. Starting at the decimal point of 0.0096 place the first digit of the answer under the first group that contains a significant number, then the second digit of the answer is placed under the next group to the right and so on. A zero is placed under any group of two zeros as follows: 0.00/96/ . The answer would then be 0.098. A quick check could be
    0   98
made by multiplying 0.09 $\times$ 0.09 = 0.0081, proving the answer in the correct range of decimal point. To try a very small number find the square root of 0.000004120. First divide into groups 0.00/00/04/12, and since there is one number in the first group with a significant figure, set 412 on the left side of the A scale, reading 2032 on the D scale. Set up the original figure as 0.00/00/04/12/00/00 with the answer below the groups. The correct square root
    0   0   2   0   3   2
is then 0.002032; to check the value 0.002 $\times$ 0.002 = 0.000004.

EXERCISES

		Trial Check
E.	The square root of 66 = 812	8 $\times$ 8 = 64
F.	The square root of 567 = 238	20 $\times$ 20 = 400

G. The square root of 0.0435 = 2085   0.2 X 0.2 = 0.04

H. The square root of 6.5 = 255   2 X 2 = 4

I. The square root of 0.000168 = 1298   0.01 X 0.01 = 0.0001

J. The square root of 5120 = 717   70 X 70 = 4900

3.8 CONVERSION AND PROPORTION

In the laboratory we use almost exclusively the metric system for units of length, weight and volume. In the home and supermarket units of measurement differ from those used in the laboratory, and we are often called upon to convert one unit to another. For example, the relation between a few common units of measurement are shown in the following list.

> 1 inch = 2.54 centimeters (1 cm = 0.3937 in)
> 1 yard = 0.9144 meters (1 m = 1.094 yd)
> 1 mile = 1.609 kilometers (1 km = 0.6214 mi)
> 1 fluid ounce = 29.57 milliliters (1 ml = 0.0338 oz)
> 1 gallon = 3.785 liters (1 1 = 0.2641 gal.)
> 1 grain = 64.8 milligrams (1 mg = 0.01543 gr)
> 1 pound = 453.6 grams (1 g = 0.002205 lb)

To convert inches to centimeters set the 1 on either end of the C scale over the 2.54 on the D scale. Then set the hairline over the required number of inches and read the answer in centimeters on the D scale. For example, 4 in = _____ cm? Set the 1 on the right side of the C scale over 2.54 on the D scale, move the hairline to 4 on the C scale and read 10.16 cm on the D scale. The speedometer on an American automobile read 60 mi/h on a British highway. What was the automobile's rate of speed in km/h? Set the 1 on the left side of the C scale over the 1.609 on the D scale, move the hairline to 60 on the C scale and read 96.6 km/h on the D scale. A 1/2 pound bottle of NaCl contains how many grams of NaCl? Set the 1 on the right side of the C scale over 453.6 on the D scale, move the hairline to 5 (0.5) on the C scale and read 226.8 g on the D scale. In general, when you set the 1 on either end of the C scale over a conversion factor, all the values on the C scale are in the units represented by the conversion factor, and all the values on the D scale are in the units to which you are converting.

EXERCISES

Convert:

A. 23.5 in to cm

B. 5 yd to m

C. 0.3 oz to ml

D. 5 gr to mg

E. 120 lb to kg

Proportions are similar to conversions, but in proportions set conversion factors are usually not given. A statement may be made that 5 yd are equivalent to 4.57 m; the question may then be asked, what is the equivalent in meters to 1.5 yd? A proportion could be set up:

$$5:4.57 = 1.5:X \text{ or } \frac{5}{4.57} = \frac{1.5}{X}$$

Solving for X

$$X = \frac{4.57 \times 1.5}{5}$$

The value X in a proportion can always be solved for by multiplication and division, as in a regular problem, or the slide rule can be used in a simplified scheme. The proportion may be set up on the C and D scales as

$$C:D = C:D \text{ or as } \frac{C}{D} = \frac{C}{D}$$

For the example 5:4.57=1.5:X, set 5 on the C scale over 4.57 on the D scale and move the hairline to 1.5 on the C scale, reading the answer 1.368 yd on the D scale. Or a problem may be stated that 3 in equal 76.2 mm; how many inches are there in 300 mm? This proportion would be set up as:

$$3:76.2 = X:300 \text{ or } \frac{3}{76.2} = \frac{X}{300}$$

Again C:D = C:D or C/D = C/D; therefore, set 3 on the C scale over 76.2 on the D scale and move the hairline to 300 on the D scale, reading the answer 11.82

in, on the C scale. If the second value on the D scale does not occur under the sliding C scale and thus cannot be read directly as in the proportion 3:76.2 = X:200, again set 3 on the C scale over the 76.2 on the D scale and observe that 200 is not under the sliding C scale. To complete the proportion set the hairline on the 1 on the left of the C scale over 254 on the D scale, move the 1 on the right of the C scale to the hairline, then move the hairline to 200 on the D scale and read the answer 7.88 in on the C scale.

You may have observed that in every proportion we are merely setting up the slide rule directly as the proportion stated. From the proportion C/D = C/D we transfer to the two scales of the slide rule: .

$$
\begin{array}{c}
C \\ D
\end{array}
\quad
\begin{array}{c}
11.82 \\ \hline 300
\end{array}
\quad
\begin{array}{c}
(X) \\ {}
\end{array}
\quad
\begin{array}{c}
3 \\ \hline 76.2
\end{array}
\quad
\begin{array}{c}
C \\ D
\end{array}
$$

OR

$$
\begin{array}{c}
C \\ D
\end{array}
\quad
\begin{array}{c}
7.88 \\ \hline 200
\end{array}
\quad
\begin{array}{c}
(X) \\ {}
\end{array}
\quad
\begin{array}{c}
3 \\ \hline 76.2
\end{array}
\quad
\begin{array}{c}
C \\ D
\end{array}
$$

OR

$$
\begin{array}{c}
C \\ D
\end{array}
\quad
\begin{array}{cc}
3 & 35.45 \ (X) \\ \hline 76.2 & 900
\end{array}
\quad
\begin{array}{c}
C \\ D
\end{array}
$$

EXERCISES

F. If 10 lb = 4.54 kg, how many lb = 50 kg?

G. If 5 mi = 8.045 km, 8 mi = how many km?

H. 9:20 = 5:X˙

I. 14:56 = X:3

J. 90:75 = X:25

3.9 THE CIRCULAR SLIDE RULE

A circular slide rule of reasonable size — for example the Dietzen Binary Slide Rule, which is 8 inches in diameter — has some distinct advantages over the common 10 inch long slide rule. The most **important advantage** is **the extra length of the commonly used scales.** The C scale used in the majority of calculations is just over 25 inches long and the L, or log scale, is almost 19 inches long. This facilitates setting of the hairline indicators and increases the accuracy of the calculations. Some idea of the advantage of a 25 inch C scale can be obtained from a study of the subdivisions of the major numbers on the scale. The largest space between 1 and 2 is not only divided into tenths, but each tenth is divided into 20 divisions, or a total of 200 divisions, with each individual division larger than one of the 100 divisions between 1 and 2 on the 10 inch long slide rule. Numbers from 2 to 5 are divided into tenths with each tenth further divided into tenths, while numbers from 5 to 10 are divided into tenths with each tenth further divided into fifths. In addition all the 100 tenths divisions between 1 and 10 are identified with a printed number corresponding to the particular tenth between any two numbers.

The front side of the slide rule has the C scale on the periphery or outer scale; under it is the C1 or inverted C scale. Then comes the A scale for squares and square roots, next the K scale for cubes and cube roots, and the fifth scale in from the periphery is the L or log scale. There are two plastic hairline indicators on the front side of the slide rule. The **long indicator** is referred to as **L**, while the **short indicator** is called **S**. It will be noted that **whenever S is moved L remains stationary**, but that **when L is moved, S moves with it**. Whenever L is moved in solving a problem be sure that nothing interferes with the free movement of S. **L always gives the answer to the problem.**

Multiplication. To multiply 1.5 × 2, first set L at 1.5 and S at 10. Turn L until S is at 2 and L will indicate the answer, 3. The new positions of L and S after moving S to 2 are indicated as L′ and S′ in the diagram. Practice multiplication by working the following problems.

EXERCISES

    A. 185 × 4.46 = _____

    B. 92 × 6.85 = _____

To multiply more than two numbers you merely repeat the simple process outlined above, as in the problem, 3 × 6 × 7. Set L at 3 and S at 10. Turn L counterclockwise until S is at 6 (answer 18). Then move S back to 10 and once again move L counterclockwise until S is at 7; read the answer 126 under the L indicator. Practice this technique with the following problems.

EXERCISES

Approximate answer

    C. 7.2 × 0.923 × 11.4 = 8 × 1 × 10 = 80

Approximate Answer

D.   52.1 × 18.9 × 5.7 × 9.3 = 50 × 20 × 5 × 10 = 50,000

Division.   To divide 3/2, first set L at 3 and S at 2. These positions are indicated as L' and S' in the diagram. Turn L' until S' is at 10 and L will indicate the answer, 1.5. Practice division by working the following problems.

FIGURE 3.8

EXERCISES

Approximate answer

E. $\dfrac{111.6}{9.7}$ $=\dfrac{100}{10}=10$

F. $\dfrac{5280}{3.141}$ $=\dfrac{5000}{3}=1667$

Combination Multiplication and Division Problems. The simplest way to solve combination type problems on a circular slide rule is to carry out **alternate, divisions and multiplications.** As an example, solve the problem $\dfrac{4 \times 30 \times 8}{6 \times 5}$. First divide 4 by 6 by setting L on 4 and S on 6 and turning L until S is at 10; then multiply the answer 0.667 by 30 by turning L until S is at 30. Next divide the answer 20 by 5 by setting S on 5 and turning until S is at 10. Finally multiply the answer 4 by 8 by turning L until S is at 8, giving the final answer 32.

After you are familiar with the circular slide rule you will discover an important shortcut in these combination problems. Let us try the short version; divide 4 by 6 by setting L on 4 and S on 6; then instead of returning S to 10, multiply by 30 by turning L until S is at 30. Next divide the answer 20 by 5 by setting S on 5; then again instead of returning S to 10, multiply by 8 by turning L until S is at 8, giving the final answer 32 at L. An extra long problem such as $\dfrac{4.25 \times 6.3 \times 22.8 \times 19.7}{0.52 \times 11.3 \times 8.8}$ could be solved by the shorter method as follows: First divide 4.25 by 0.52 by setting L on 4.25 and S on 0.52; then multiply by 6.3 by turning L until S is at 6.3. Next divide the answer (51.5) on L by 11.3 by setting S on 11.3; then multiply by 22.8 by turning L until S is at 22.8. Finally divide the answer (104.0) on L by 8.8 by setting S on 8.8, then multiply by 19.7 by turning L until S is at 19.7, giving the answer 232.8. Practice the short method by solving the following problems.

EXERCISES

Approximate Answer

G. $\dfrac{33 \times 5 \times 3}{9 \times 2}$ $=\dfrac{30 \times 5 \times 3}{10 \times 2}=22.5$

H. $\dfrac{68.3 \times 3.141 \times 11.2}{5.67 \times 9.12}$ $=\dfrac{70 \times 3 \times 10}{5 \times 10}=42$

Square and Square Roots. The technique of finding the square or square root of a number is exactly the same as on a 10 inch slide rule. The C and A scales (first and third) are used on the circular slide rule. Set L on any number on the C scale and read the square under the hairline on the A scale. For example, square 6.89 = 7 × 7 = 49, correct answer 47.5. In solving square root problems, if the answer is 1 or greater, space off groups of two digits from the decimal point to your left. If the last group to the left has one digit, use the first half of the A scale; if the last group to the left has two digits, use the last half of the A scale. As an example, to find the square root of 450.0 space off two digits to the left and find one digit in the last group (4/50.0). Setting 450.0 on the first half of A, find 212 on the C scale. Since 20 × 20 = 400 the correct answer is 21.2. If the number is less than 1, space off groups of two digits from the decimal point to your right. If the first group with a significant figure to the right of the decimal point contains one number, use the first half of the A scale; if the group contains two numbers, use the second half of the A scale. The square root of 0.000860 would be obtained by dividing into groups as 0.00/08/60, and since there is one number in the first group with a significant figure, set 860 on the first half of the A scale, reading 293 on the C scale. Set up the original figure as 0.00/08/60/00 with the answer below the groups, as with the 10 inch slide rule.

     0   2   9   3

The correct square root is then 0.0293; to check the value, 0.03 × 0.03 = 0.0009.

EXERCISES

Trial check

I. The square root of 73 = 854   8 × 8 = 64

J. The square root of 0.00445 = 667   0.07 × 0.07 = 0.0049

Conversion and Proportion. The main difference between conversion and proportion problems on the circular slide rule is the technique of setting the scales and reading the answers to the problems. A few examples utilizing the circular slide rule will suffice to make the point. To convert 6 inches to centimeters with the relationship 1 in = 2.54 cm set L on 2.54 and S on 10; then move L until S is at 6, and L will indicate the answer, 15.24 cm. A 5 pound bottle of glucose contains how many grams of glucose? Since 1 lb = 453.6 g, set L on 453.6 and S on 10; then move L until S is at 5, and L will indicate the answer, 2268 g. Proportions are simple to calculate once the proportion is correctly set up. If 8 yd is equivalent to 7.32 m, how many meters are equivalent to 2.5 yd? The proportion could be set up as:

$$8:7.32 = 2.5:X \text{ or } \frac{8}{7.32} = \frac{2.5}{X} \text{ or } X = \frac{7.32 \times 2.5}{8}$$

A simple division followed by a multiplication would be solved as follows: Divide 7.32 by 8 by setting L on 7.32 and S on 8; then multiply by 2.5 by turning L until S is at 2.5, reading the answer, 2.287, meters on L.

EXERCISES

K. If 20 lb = 9.09 kg, how many lb = 70 kg?

L. 95:80 = X:32

M. If 60 mi = 96.54 km, 150 mi = how many kilometers?

ADDITIONAL EXERCISES

1. Carry out the following calculations with a slide rule.

a. 220 × 13

b. 3.3 × 69

c. 96.2 × 4.5 × 21.3

d. 22.2 × 316 × 42.4

e. 6.1 × 11.5 × 206 × 96.8

2. Work the following problems with a slide rule.

a. $\dfrac{5280}{3}$

b. $\dfrac{5 \times 21 \times 9}{7 \times 2}$

c. $\dfrac{17.5 \times 110.1 \times 68}{51.6 \times 22.2}$

d. $\dfrac{0.198 \times 98.8 \times 12.3}{0.202 \times 53.1}$

e. $\dfrac{3.14 \times 5280 \times 1.5 \times 9.9}{23.1 \times 2.2 \times 8.5}$

3. Calculate the following with a slide rule.

    a. 31.3^2

    b. 1.51^2

    c. $\sqrt{552}$

    d. $\sqrt{0.056}$

    e. $\sqrt{67.5}$

4. Convert the following units.

    a. 141 in to cm

    b. 36 in to cm

    c. 200 lb to kg

    d. 130 lb to kg

    e. 10 gr to mg

    f. 1.25 gr to mg

    g. 60 mi to km

    h. 8 oz to ml

5. Calculate the following proportions:

    a. 80:20 = X:10

    b. If 50 lb = 22.7 kg, how many pounds = 50 kg?

c. If 5 gr = 324 mg, how many grains = 500 mg?

d. If 176.0 yd = 0.1 mi, how many yards = 5 mi?

e. If 2 oz = 59.14 ml, how many ounces = 1000 ml?

4
Concentration of Solutions

THE *PRACTICAL OBJECTIVES* OF THIS CHAPTER ARE TO OBTAIN AN UNDERSTANDING OF:

1. Basic S.I. units and their prefixes for multiple and submultiple units.
2. The fundamental difference between percentage, molar, and normal solutions.
3. The use of the simple relation between volume and concentration in dilution and conversion problems.

In the preceding sections we have been exposed to, and in some instances reviewed, the expression of numbers, powers of ten, roots, logarithms and the use of the slide rule. If you are willing to thoughtfully practice the examples that were given to enable you to **become proficient in arithmetical common sense** and in the use of logarithms and the slide rule, you will possess the tools **to solve any of the problems in laboratory mathematics.**

There are many occasions in the laboratory when it is necessary for the technician to prepare solutions to be used in routine or research methods and reactions. Obviously it is important that every solution be correctly prepared, and to complete such an assignment you must first understand the expressions of concentration and then be able to correctly calculate the quantities of solvent and solute required to make the solution.

4.1 INTERNATIONAL SYSTEM OF UNITS AND QUANTITIES

The **international system of units** called S.I. is an attempt to attain uniformity among all scientific disciplines in the expression of results from experimental data. Wherever practical we should attempt to use this system of units and quantities in the preparation of solutions and the expression of their concentrations. As you will soon learn, there are expressions of concentration such as percentage solutions and milliequivalents per liter of electrolytes that have not as yet been replaced by S.I. units. Basic quantities and units that apply in practical laboratory calculations are listed in Table 4.1.

TABLE 4.1 BASIC S.I. UNITS AND QUANTITIES

Basic Unit of	Name	Symbol	Other Common Units	
Length	meter	m	millimeter, mm	nanometer, nm
Mass	kilogram	kg	gram, g	milligram, mg
Volume	cubic meter	m³	liter, l milliliter, ml	deciliter, dl microliter, μl
Time	second	s	minute, min day, d	hour, h day, 24 h
Amount of substance	mole	M	millimole, mM	micromole, μM
Concentration	kilogram/liter	kg/l	milligrams/ 100 ml	milligrams/ deciliter, mg/dl

A series of common prefixes for multiples and submultiples of the **S.I. units** will be found very helpful in the expression of terms and calculations involving these units (Table 4.2)

TABLE 4.2 PREFIXES FOR S.I. UNITS

Multiple	Prefix	Symbol	Multiple	Prefix	Symbol
10^{12}	tera	T	10^{-3}	milli	m
10^{9}	giga	G	10^{-6}	micro	μ
10^{6}	mega	M	10^{-9}	nano	n
10^{3}	kilo	k	10^{-12}	pico	p
			10^{-15}	femto	f

4.2 PERCENTAGE SOLUTIONS

Per cent means parts per hundred and is commonly used by banks as per cent interest. If the banks pay 5 per cent interest per year on savings, a deposit of $100 would earn $5 interest in one year. In the laboratory per cent is expressed as grams per hundred or milliliters per hundred. The three most common percentage solutions used in the laboratory are:

1. grams of solute in 100 milliliters of solution (W/V)

  2. grams of solute in 100 grams of solution (W/W)

  3. milliliters of liquid in 100 milliliters of solution (V/V)

W/V signifies weight per volume, W/W weight per weight and V/V volume per volume. In most laboratories the **weight per volume solutions** are used because the solute is important and the solvent is merely used as the vehicle for the solute. The physical chemist prefers to weigh both the solute and solvent to prepare weight per weight solutions because the concentration does not change with changes in temperature. The volume per volume solutions are the least accurate and are used when the solute is a liquid, as in alcohol solutions.

The preparation of a 5 per cent solution of sodium chloride, for example, on a weight per volume basis would consist of dissolving 5 g of sodium chloride in water and then diluting the solution to a final volume of 100 ml. On a weight per weight basis, 5 g of sodium chloride would be added to 95 g of water and dissolved to form 100 g of solution. A solution of two liquids on a volume per volume basis, as, for example, a 10 per cent solution of alcohol, would be prepared by adding 10 ml of alcohol to water and diluting to a final volume of 100 ml. In simple calculations involving percentage solutions first determine the quantity of solute contained in 100 ml of solution. It then becomes relatively easy to calculate the quantity of solute present in a given volume.

Examples

Find the weight of glucose that must be used to prepare 800 ml of a 5 per cent solution. First we can state that a 5 per cent solution contains 5 g of glucose in 100 ml of solvent. Since 800 ml is required 800/100 = 8 times the amount in 100 ml or 8 X 5 = 40 g of glucose that must be used to prepare 800 ml of a 5 per cent solution.

What volume of isotonic saline (0.85% NaCl) can be prepared from 42.5 g of NaCl? In outline form:

1. An 0.85 per cent solution contains 0.85 g in 100 ml.

2. Since 42.5 g are to be used, $\dfrac{42.5}{0.85}$ = 50 times the amount in 100 ml.

3. 50 X 100 ml = 5000 ml of 0.85 per cent NaCl solution contains the 42.5 g.

A weighed quantity of NaCl (50.0 g) was accidently transferred to a beaker containing approximately 200 ml of distilled water. How would you proceed to prepare a 5 per cent NaCl solution from the contents of the beaker?

1. A 5 per cent solution contains 5 g in 100 ml.

2. Since 50 g NaCl are in the beaker, $\frac{50}{5}$ = 10 times the amount in 100 ml.

3. 10 X 100 ml = 1000 ml of 5 per cent NaCl solution equivalent to 50 g.

4. Quantitatively transfer the NaCl solution from the beaker to a liter volumetric flask and dilute to the 1000 ml mark with water.

EXERCISES

A. Find the weight of sodium sulfate that must be used to prepare 250 ml of a 23 per cent solution.

B. A saturated solution of potassium chloride contains 34.7 g in 100 ml of solution at 20°C. How many grams of potassium chloride must be added to 500 ml of a 10 per cent solution to saturate the solution at 20°C? (Disregard changes in volume caused by addition of solid KCl.)

Before proceeding to problems that involve molar or normal solutions and even before discussing more complicated percentage solutions we must consider a few accessory points such as specific gravity of solutions and inorganic salts having varying numbers of molecules of water of hydration.

4.3 SPECIFIC GRAVITY

The density of both solids and liquids is usually expressed in grams per milliliter (g/ml). The density of mercury, for example, is 13.6 g/ml, meaning of course that each milliliter of mercury weighs 13.6 grams. The **specific gravity** of a solid or liquid is a number that expresses the ratio of the weight of the solid or liquid to the weight of an equal volume of water at 4°C taken as a standard.

$$\text{Specific gravity} = \frac{\text{Weight of solid or liquid}}{\text{Weight of an equal volume of water at } 4°C}$$

The density of water changes very little between 4° and 30°C; therefore, the value 1.00 g/ml may be used as a standard for specific gravity measurements at ordinary laboratory temperatures. The specific gravity of a solid or liquid is the same when any system of units is used, because it expresses the ratio of the weight of the solid or liquid to the weight of an equal volume of water. Specific gravity values are therefore expressed as a number without any units. For example, the specific gravity of normal urine varies from 1.008 to 1.030.

Examples

Find the density and specific gravity of ethyl alcohol if 8.0 ml weighs 6.40 g.

1. If 8.0 ml weighs 6.4 g, then 1 ml weighs $\dfrac{6.4}{8.0}$ = 0.80 g.

2. The density is therefore 0.80 g/ml and the specific gravity is
$$\dfrac{0.80 \text{ g/ml}}{1.00 \text{ g/ml}(H_2O)} = 0.80$$

A volume of urine (500 ml) weighs 510.0 g. What is the specific gravity of the urine specimen?

Since 500 ml of urine weighs 510 g and 500 ml of water weighs 500 g,

$\dfrac{510}{500}$ = 1.020, the specific gravity of the urine.

Concentrated sulfuric acid contains 98 per cent H_2SO_4 by weight and has a specific gravity of 1.84. How many grams of H_2SO_4 are there in 400 ml of concentrated acid?

One milliliter of concentrated acid contains $0.98 \times 1.84 = 1.80$ g H_2SO_4; therefore 400 ml of concentrated H_2SO_4 contains $400 \times 1.80 = 720$ g of H_2SO_4.

EXERCISES

A. What would be the volume of 20 kg of a glycerol solution that had a specific gravity of 1.55?

B. A small volume, 25 ml, of a heavy liquid weighs 340 g. What is the specific gravity of the liquid?

C. Concentrated hydrochloric acid contains 37.5 per cent HCl by weight and has a specific gravity of 1.19. Calculate the weight of HCl in 10.0 ml of concentrated hydrochloric acid.

4.4 HYDRATES AND WATER OF HYDRATION

In addition to anhydrous salts you will often find reagent bottles of hydrated solid inorganic salts, as, for example, $CuSO_4 \cdot 5 H_2O$, $BaCl_2 \cdot 2 H_2O$, and so on. When preparing solutions we usually weigh quantities of the solid solute to be dissolved in a definite volume of final solution.

To prepare a 5 per cent solution of $CuSo_4$ when only the hydrate $CuSO_4 \cdot 5 H_2O$ is available, we must calculate the weight of the hydrate that contains 5 g of $CuSo_4$ (anhydrous). This is accomplished by dividing the formula weight of $CuSO_4 \cdot 5 H_2O$ by the formula weight of $CuSO_4$ and multiplying by 5, as follows:

$$\frac{CuSO_4 \cdot 5 H_2O}{CuSO_4} = \frac{63.5 + 32 + 64 + 10 + 80}{63.5 + 32 + 64} = \frac{249.5}{159.5} \times 5 = 7.83 \text{ g.}$$

It would be necessary to weigh 7.83 g of $CuSO_4 \cdot 5 H_2O$ to obtain 5 g of the anhydrous salt to dissolve in water for a total volume of 100 ml of a 5 per cent solution.

Example

One pound (453.6) of $BaCl_2 \cdot H_2O$ is equivalent to what weight of $BaCl_2$?

1. 1. g of $BaCl_2 \cdot 2H_2O$ is equivalent to:

$$\frac{BaCl_2}{BaCl_2 \cdot 2 H_2O} = \frac{137.3 + 71}{137.3 + 71 + 36} = \frac{208.3}{244.3} = 0.853 \text{ g.}$$

2. $453.6 \times 0.853 = 386$ g.

3. One pound of $BaCl_2 \cdot 2 H_2O$ contains 386 g of $BaCl_2$.

EXERCISES

A. A pound of washing soda, $Na_2CO_3 \cdot 10 H_2O$, contains what percentage of water?

B. Find the weight of $Na_2SO_4 \cdot 7 H_2O$ that must be used to prepare 250 ml of a 23 per cent solution of Na_2SO_4.

4.5 MOLAR SOLUTIONS

A gram molecular weight of a substance is known as a **mole. A solution that contains 1 mole of the solute in 1 liter is called a molar solution.** The abbreviation for molar is M; thus, a one molar solution can be expressed as 1 M.

Examples

What weight of H_2SO_4 is required to prepare 400 ml of a 3 M solution?

1. The molecular weight of H_2SO_4 is 98; therefore, one liter of 3 M solution contains $3 \times 98 = 294$ g H_2SO_4 .

2. If one liter contains 294 g, 400 ml contains $0.4 \times 294 = 117.6$ g of H_2SO_4.

How many grams of NaCl would be required to prepare 600 ml of a 2.5 M solution?

1. The molecular weight of NaCl is 58.5; therefore one liter of 2.5 M solution contains $2.5 \times 58.5 = 146.25$ g NaCl.

2. If one liter contains 146.25 g, 600 ml contains $0.6 \times 146.25 = 87.75$ g of NaCl.

When working with molar solutions if you first determine the quantity of solution in a liter, it is then easy to calculate fractions or multiples of that value. In general chemistry we learned that several salts and hydroxides do not have true molecular weights. This fact makes it difficult to express all compounds in moles, although a formula may be written for any given compound. Some chemists prefer formal solutions to molar solutions and formality instead of molarity. A formal solution, abbreviated F, contains a gram formula weight in a liter of solution and in many instances is the same as a molar solution. Since it is common practice in most laboratories to express concentration in terms of molarity, we will retain the molar designation.

In the modern laboratory the use of micromethods, the study of subcellular components and the vast scope of enzyme methodology have given rise to the expressions of concentrations in **millimoles**, mM, and **micromoles**, μM. A millimole is the molecular weight in milligrams instead of grams, and micromole is a microgram molecular weight. These small concentrations are also often expressed as 1×10^{-3} M, which equals 1 mM, or 1×10^{-6} M, which equals 1 μM.

Another useful relation is the fact that **each milliliter of a 1 M solution contains 1 mM of the solute.**

Examples

How many grams of HCl would be required to prepare 500 ml of a 1×10^{-3} M solution?

1. A 1×10^{-3} M solution = 1 mM HCl solution, which contains a milligram molecular weight per liter or 36.5 mg/l.

2. If one liter contains 36.5 mg, 500 ml contains 18.25 mg, and 0.01825 g of HCl is needed to prepare 500 ml of a 1×10^{-3} M solution.

How many micrograms of NaOH would be required to prepare 250 ml of a 2×10^{-6} M solution?

1. A 1×10^{-6} M solution = 1 μM NaOH solution, which contains a microgram molecular weight per liter, or 40 μg/l.

2. One liter of 2×10^{-6} would then contain 2×40 μg/l = 80 μg NaOH/l.

3. If one liter contains 80 μg, 250 ml contains $0.25 \times 80 = 20$ μg of NaOH.

EXERCISES

A. What weight of NaOH is required to prepare 3000 ml of a 0.5 M solution?

B. How many micrograms of NaCl would 300 ml of a 1×10^{-6} M solution contain?

C. A solution contains 3.65 g of HCl in a liter. How many millimoles of HCl does it contain?

4.6 MOLAL SOLUTIONS

A molal solution contains 1 mole of the solute in 1000 g of solvent. In comparison, a molar solution has a final volume of 1000 ml, whereas the volume of a molal solution exceeds 1000 ml. Physical chemists often use molal solutions because temperature changes do not affect the concentration as they do in molar solutions. Most laboratories do not weigh the solvent and also do not require the exacting properties of molal solutions in their reactions. We shall not, therefore, give examples of the preparation or calculation of molal solutions.

4.7 NORMAL SOLUTIONS

A normal solution contains one gram equivalent weight of the solute in 1 liter of solution. A gram equivalent weight is the quantity of a substance that will replace or react with 1.008 g of hydrogen. The gram equivalent weight of an acid would be the weight equivalent to 1.008 g of replaceable hydrogen. An equivalent weight of a base is the weight that combines with 1.008 g of replaceable hydrogen. For example, 1 mole of HCl (36.5 g), 1/2 mole of H_2SO_4 (49 g), 1 mole of NaOH (40 g), 1/3 mole of $Al(OH)_3$ (26 g), and 1/2 mole of K_2SO_4 (87 g), each in 1 liter of solution would represent normal solutions of these compounds. A one normal solution is abbreviated 1 N solution. Since a milligram equivalent weight of a substance would be a milliequivalent, a normal solution of a compound would contain 1 milliequivalent of solute in 1 ml of solution. A tabulation of the approximate normality and ml/l required to prepare a 1 N solution from concentrated solutions of the common acids and bases may be found in the Appendix.

Examples

How many milliliters of concentrated HCl (specific gravity 1.19 and 37.50 per cent HCl by weight) would be required to prepare 15 l of 0.1 N acid?

1. The equivalent weight of $HCl = \dfrac{36.5}{1} = 36.5$; therefore, 1 liter of 0.1 N solution contains $\dfrac{36.5}{10} = 3.65$ g HCl and 15 l would contain 15 × 3.65 = 54.75 g.

2. One milliliter of concentrated acid contains 0.375 × 1.19 = 0.446 g HCl. Therefore, 15 liters of 0.1 N HCl requires $\dfrac{54.75}{0.446} = 122.8$ ml of concentrated acid.

How many milliequivalents of a solute are contained in 500 ml of a 3 N solution?

One liter (1000 ml) of a 1 N solution contains 1000 milliequivalents; therefore, 1000 ml of a 3 N solution contains 3 × 1000 or 3000 milliequivalents and 500 ml contains $\dfrac{3000}{2}$ = 1500 milliequivalents in 500 ml of a 3 N solution.

What weight of $Al(OH)_3$ is required to prepare 2.5 liters of a 0.1 N solution?

1. The equivalent weight of $Al(OH)_3$ is 26; therefore, one liter of 0.1 N solution contains 0.1 X 26 = 2.6 g $Al(OH)_3$.

2. If one liter contains 2.6 g, 2.5 liters contains 2.5 X 2.6 = 6.5 g $Al(OH)_3$.

EXERCISES

A. How many milliliters of concentrated sulfuric acid (specific gravity 1.84 and 98 per cent H_2SO_4 by weight) are required to prepare 3 l of 0.2 N solution?

B. What is the normality of isotonic saline (0.85 per cent NaCl)?

C. Given 500 ml of a 40 per cent solution of NaOH, to what volume of 1 N NaOH is this equivalent?

4.8 DILUTION OF SOLUTIONS

All of the solutions that we have previously considered are known as volumetric solutions and all contain a definite amount of solute in a fixed volume of solution. In percentage, molar, molal or normal solutions, the amount of solute contained in a given volume of solution is equal to the product of the volume times the concentration. When a solution is diluted, its volume is increased and its concentration is decreased; however, the total amount of solute remains unchanged. Two solutions with different concentrations that contain the same amount of solute can therefore be related to each other as follows:

$$\text{Amount of solute}_1 = \text{Volume}_1 \times \text{Concentration}_1$$
$$\text{Amount of solute}_2 = \text{Volume}_2 \times \text{Concentration}_2$$

Since the amount of solute$_1$ = amount of solute $_2$, then:

$$\textbf{Volume}_1 \times \textbf{Concentration}_1 = \textbf{Volume}_2 \times \textbf{Concentration}_2$$

If the volume and concentration on both sides of the equation are expressed in the same units, this relationship will apply in many calculations. For example:

$$ml \times N = ml \times N$$

$$l \times M = l \times M$$

$$ml \times \mu M = ml \times \mu M$$

Examples

How much water should be added to 2 l of 0.12 N hydrochloric acid to prepare a solution of 0.10 N HCl?

From the equation:
$$ml_1 \times N_1 = ml_2 \times N_2$$
Let X = volume of 0.10 N solution (ml_1)
$$X_{ml} \times 0.10 \text{ N} = 2000 \text{ ml} \times 0.12 \text{ N}$$
or $X = \dfrac{2000 \times 0.12}{0.10} = 2400$ ml of 0.10 N HCl and 2400 − 2000 (the 2000 ml of 0.12 N) = 400 ml of water that should be added to the 2 l of 0.12 N HCl to prepare 0.10 N HCl.

What volume of 10 per cent NaCl solution would be required to prepare 800 ml of a 0.85 per cent solution?

From the equation:
$$ml_1 \times \text{per cent}_1 = ml_2 \times \text{per cent}_2$$
Let X = volume of 10 per cent solution (ml_1)
$$X_{ml} \times 10 \text{ per cent} = 800 \text{ ml} \times 0.85 \text{ per cent}$$
or $X = \dfrac{800 \times 0.85}{10} = 68$ ml of 10 per cent NaCl required.

A stock solution of 2.5 M $NaHCO_3$ is available. How many milliliters of the stock solution should be diluted to 100 ml to prepare a 25 mM $NaHCO_3$ standard?

From the equation $ml_1 \times mM_1 = ml_2 \times mM_2$, express 2.5 M in millimolar concentration = 2500 mM.

Let X = volume of 2.5 M $NaHCO_3$
X ml × 2500 mM = 100 ml × 25 mM, or
$$X = \dfrac{100 \times 25}{2500} = 1.0$$ ml of stock solution diluted to 100 ml.

EXERCISES

A. Given 50 ml of a 12 μM solution of $BaCl_2$, what volume of 3 μM $BaCl_2$ could be prepared from this solution?

B. Fifteen liters of approximately 0.1 N NaOH were prepared from a stock solution. An accurate titration indicated a normality of 0.1055 N. How much water should be added to the 15 liters to prepare 0.100 N NaOH?

C. What volume of a stock solution of 20 per cent phosphoric acid would be required to prepare 600 ml of a 1.5 per cent solution?

In the clinical laboratory dilutions that are commonly encountered are the **dilution of a specimen** for accurate analysis and the **dilution of a standard** to correspond to the concentration in the serum. These dilutions are expressed as a ratio, such as 1:10, which refers to 1 unit of the original solution diluted to a final volume of 10 units. The diluted solution would be 1/10 the concentration of the original solution, and its concentration would be calculated by multiplying the concentration of the original solution by the dilution expressed as a fraction.

Examples

A 100 mg/100 ml glucose solution is diluted 1:5. What is the concentration of the dilute solution?

Original solution = 100 mg/100 ml × the dilution 1/5 = 20 mg/100 ml

A serum specimen was diluted 1:2, and this diluted solution was further diluted 1:4. If the concentration of the final diluted solution was 50 mg/100 ml, what was the concentration in the serum specimen? To calculate the original concentration we must reverse the dilution fractions:

$$50 \text{ mg}/100 \text{ ml} \times \frac{2}{1} \times \frac{4}{1} = 400 \text{ mg}/100 \text{ ml serum concentration}$$

To check: $400 \text{ mg}/100 \text{ ml} \times \frac{1}{2} \times \frac{1}{4} = 50 \text{ mg}/100 \text{ ml}$

Serum is often diluted 1:10 in the preparation of a protein-free filtrate. If 1 ml of the filtrate is used in a spectrophotometric method and 1 ml of a standard solution is carried through the same method, the standard solution must be diluted 1:10 if it is to represent the serum concentration. Under these conditions what standard concentration would correspond to a serum glucose level of 200 mg/100 ml? Serum diluted 1:10, so $200 \times \frac{1}{10} = 20$ mg/100 ml the concentration of the standard used in the method.

EXERCISES

D. A 500 mg/100 ml solution was diluted 1:10, and this diluted solution was further diluted 1:5. What is the concentration of the final solution?

E. A serum specimen was diluted 1:10, and this diluted solution was further diluted 1:3. If the concentration of the final diluted solution was 20 mg/100 ml, what was the concentration in the serum specimen?

4.9 CONVERSION PROBLEMS

Problems in the laboratory that involve **conversion from one unit of concentration to another** are often encountered. The preparation of normal or molar solutions from percentage solutions or the expression of mg/100 ml units as milliequivalents/liter are common conversion problems. All the principles that have been discussed under solutions will be applied to conversion problems. In general, the first step is to convert the given units to the desired units of concentration and then to calculate any dilution problem using similar units.

Examples

How many milliliters of 22 per cent Na_2SO_4 would be required to prepare 500 ml of a 0.5 M solution?

1. A 22 per cent Na_2SO_4 solution contains 22 g/100 ml $\times$ 10 = 220 g/l.

2. A 1 M Na_2SO_4 solution contains one gram molecular weight or 142 g/l. Therefore, 22 per cent $Na_2SO_4 = \frac{220 \text{ g/l}}{142 \text{ g/l}} = 1.55$ M.

3. From $ml_1 \times M_1 = ml_2 \times M_2$

Let X = volume of the 1.55 M solution, therefore

$$X_{ml} \times 1.55 \text{ M} = 500 \text{ ml} \times 0.5 \text{ M}$$

or $X = \dfrac{500 \times 0.5}{1.55} = 161.5$ ml of 22 per cent Na_2SO_4 required.

Calculate the percentage concentration of 5 N H_2SO_4.

1. The equivalent weight of H_2SO_4 is $\dfrac{98}{2} = 49$; therefore, a 5 N solution contains $5 \times 49 = 245$ g/l.

2. The $\dfrac{245 \text{ g/l}}{10} = 24.5$ g/100 ml = 24.5 per cent.

How many milliliters of 5 per cent HCl would be required to prepare 250 ml of a 0.1 N solution?

1. A 5 per cent HCl solution contains 5 g/100 ml $\times$ 10 = 50 g/l.

2. A 1 N solution contains one gram equivalent weight, or 36.5 g/l.

Therefore, 5 per cent HCl $= \dfrac{50 \text{ g/l}}{36.5 \text{ g/l}} = 1.37$ N.

3. From $ml_1 \times N_1 = ml_2 \times N_2$,

let X = volume of the 1.37 N solution.

X ml $\times$ 1.37 N = 250 ml $\times$ 0.1 N, or

$X = \dfrac{250 \times 0.1}{1.37} = 18.25$ ml of 5 per cent HCl required.

Another common conversion problem involves milliequivalents per liter. We have already seen that 1 ml of a 1 N solution contains 1 milliequivalent of a solute. Since electrolyte concentrations in body fluids are ordinarily expressed in milliequivalents per liter and many of the plasma constituents are represented in milligrams per 100 milliliters, conversion problems are involved. In general, to convert mg/100 ml to milliequivalents/l (mEq/l), we must first multiply by 10 to obtain mg/l and then divide by the equivalent weight to obtain mEq/l.

Examples

Convert 350 mg/100 ml of Na^+ to mEq/l.

1. The milligrams per liter = 350 × 10 = 3500 mg/l.

2. The mg/l divided by the equivalent weight of Na = $\dfrac{3500}{23}$ = 152.2 mEq/l.

A solution of NaCl has a concentration of 145 mEq/l. Convert this to percentage concentration.

1. Since $\dfrac{mg/l}{equiv.\ wt.}$ = mEq/l, then mg/l = mEq/l × equiv. wt. or mg/l = 145 × 58.5 = 8500 mg/l.

2. 8500 mg/l = 850 mg/100 ml = 0.85 g/100 ml = 0.85 per cent NaCl.

A patient had a serum Ca concentration of 12 mg/100 ml. Express this concentration in mEq/l.

1. The milligrams per liter = 12 × 10 = 120 mg/l.

2. The mg/l divided by the equivalent weight of Ca $\left(\dfrac{40}{2}\right)$ = $\dfrac{120}{20}$ = 6 mEq/l.

EXERCISES

A. How many milliliters of 10 per cent HCl would be required to prepare 600 ml of a 0.5 M solution?

B. Calculate the normality of:

    a. Concentrated HCl (specific gravity 1.19; 37.5 per cent HCl by weight).

    b. Concentrated H_2SO_4 (specific gravity 1.84; 98 per cent H_2SO_4 by weight).

    c. 50 per cent NaOH solution.

ADDITIONAL EXERCISES

1. A liter of 5 per cent glucose solution contains what weight of glucose?

2. A 24 hour urine specimen (1250 ml) weighed 1275 g. What is the specific gravity of the urine specimen?

3. Concentrated sulfuric acid has a specific gravity of 1.84 and is 98 per cent H_2SO_4 by weight. Calculate the weight of H_2SO_4 in 55.0 ml of concentrated sulfuric acid.

4. If you were offered 5 lb of $CuSO_4 \cdot 5H_2O$ for $5.00 and 5 lb of an-hydrous $CuSO_4$ for $7.00, which would be the best buy?

5. How many grams of H_2SO_4 would 1 liter of 1×10^{-3} M solution contain?

6. What weight of NaCl would be required to prepare 800 ml of 1 M solution?

7. A liter of 0.1 N H_2SO_4 was prepared from concentrated H_2SO_4 (specific gravity 1.84; 98 per cent by weight). How many milliliters of the concentrated acid was required?

8. Sixteen liters of approximately 0.1 N HCl were prepared from concentrated HCl. An accurate titration indicated a normality of 0.1037. How much water should be added to the 16 l to prepare 0.100 N HCl?

9. A stock solution of NaOH was exactly 12.0 N. How many milliliters of the stock solution would be used to prepare 16 l of 0.200 N NaOH?

10. Calculate the percentage concentration of 8 N HCl.

11. How many milliliters of 36.5 per cent HCl would be required to prepare 500 ml of a 5.0 N solution?

12. A patient's serum had a NaCl concentration of 609 mg/100 ml. What would the concentration of NaCl be in mEq/l?

5
Hydrogen Ion Concentration and pH

THE *PRACTICAL OBJECTIVES* OF THIS CHAPTER ARE TO OBTAIN AN UNDERSTANDING OF:

1. The ionization of strong and weak acids and their hydrogen ion concentrations.

2. The approximation and accurate calculation of pH values.

3. The conversion of the pH of a solution to its hydrogen ion concentration.

In biological fluids, which are essentially water solutions, an acid may be defined as a substance that yields protons and a base as a substance that accepts protons. From a more practical standpoint, in an aqueous solution an **acid** may be regarded as a substance that **yields hydrogen ions** $(\overset{+}{H})$ and a **base** as a substance that **yields hydroxide ions** $(\overline{OH})$. When an acid or base is added to water, the degree of dissociation into ions will determine the relative strength of the acid or basic solution. In a dilute solution a **strong acid** such as HCl will dissociate almost completely into $(\overset{+}{H})$ and $(\overline{Cl})$ ions. **A weak acid,** such as acetic acid, under the same conditions will dissociate only slightly into $(\overset{+}{H})$ and (CH_3COO) ions. Assuming 100 per cent ionization of HCl and 1 per cent ionization of acetic acid in 0.1 N solution, the $[\overset{+}{H}]$ concentration could be calculated as follows:

$$N \times \% \text{ ionization} = [\overset{+}{H}] \text{ concentration}$$

For HCl $\qquad$ 0.1 N $\times$ 1.00 (100%) = 0.100 = $[\overset{+}{H}]$

For acetic acid $\qquad$ 0.1 N $\times$ 0.01 $\quad$ (1%) = 0.001 = $[\overset{+}{H}]$

Water dissociates very slightly into $(\overset{+}{H})$ and $(\overline{OH})$ ions as follows:

$$H_2O \rightleftharpoons \overset{+}{H} + \overline{OH}$$

It can be shown that 10,000,000 liters of water will yield 1 g of $(\overset{+}{H})$, or that one liter of water contains 1/10,000,000 of a gram of hydrogen ions. The **hydrogen**

ion concentration of water therefore equals $\frac{1}{10^7}$ or 10^{-7} g/l. The hydrogen ion and hydroxide ion concentrations of water must be equal since water is a neutral solution. The $[\overset{+}{H}]$ concentration = 10^{-7} and the $[\overline{OH}]$ concentration = 10^{-7} and the dissociation constant, K_W, for water equals

$$K_W = 10^{-7} \times 10^{-7} = 10^{-14}$$

Since a neutral solution such as water has a hydrogen ion concentration of 10^{-7}, it follows that an acid solution must have a $[\overset{+}{H}]$ concentration greater than 10^{-7} and that a basic solution must have a $[\overset{+}{H}]$ concentration less than 10^{-7}.

In 1909, Sorensen decided that laboratory workers would experience difficulty in expressing $[\overset{+}{H}]$ concentrations of acid and basic solutions in terms of exponential numbers. He devised the term **pH**, which he defined as **the negative logarithm of the $[\overset{+}{H}]$ concentration.** The relation is exceedingly simple if the $[\overset{+}{H}]$ concentration is exactly $1 \times 10^{-\text{power}}$ because the pH then equals the value of the negative power of ten. For example, water has a hydrogen ion concentration of 10^{-7}, or a pH of 7; the 0.1 N HCl from the example above has a $[\overset{+}{H}]$ concentration of 0.1, or 10^{-1}, or a pH of 1; and the 0.1 N acetic acid with a $[\overset{+}{H}]$ concentration of 0.001, or 10^{-3}, has a pH of 3. To calculate the pH of a solution with a $[\overset{+}{H}]$ concentration more complex than $1 \times 10^{-\text{power}}$ we must resort to the use of logarithms as follows:

$$pH = \log \frac{1}{[\overset{+}{H}]} = -\log [\overset{+}{H}]$$

Since the $[\overset{+}{H}]$ is expressed as a $\times 10^{-b}$ the pH = $-\log a \times 10^{-b}$ or pH = b $-\log$ a. If the $[\overset{+}{H}]$ concentration of a solution is 0.004, calculate the pH.

Example

$$\text{The } [\overset{+}{H}] = a \times 10^{-b} = 4 \times 10^{-3}$$

The pH = $-\log 4 \times 10^{-3}$ or $3 - \log 4$ as (b $-\log$ a)

Calculating, $3 - \log 4 = 3 - 0.602 = 2.398 = $ pH

The pH value for any $[\overset{+}{H}]$ concentration can be approximated mentally by expressing the $[\overset{+}{H}]$ concentration between 1×10 to a negative power and 10×10 to the same negative power. For example, 0.005 can be expressed as 5×10^{-3} and falls between 1×10^{-3} and 10×10^{-3}. The pH corresponding to

$1 \times 10^{-3} = 3$ and to $10 \times 10^{-3} = 1 \times 10^{-2} = 2$. If the logarithm scale were linear, we would estimate 5×10^{-3} as a pH of 2.5, however a quick study of the approximate logarithms of values from 1 to 9 will yield a more accurate estimate. This method of approximation is illustrated in the following tabulation:

TABLE 5.1   APPROXIMATION OF pH VALUES

Number $\times 10^{-power}$ $(a \times 10^{-b})$	Approximate Logarithm	$(\overset{+}{H})$ Concentration	Approximate pH $(b - \log a)$
1	0	1×10^{-3}	3.0
2	0.3	2×10^{-3}	2.7
3	0.5	3×10^{-3}	2.5
4	0.6	4×10^{-3}	2.4
5	0.7	5×10^{-3}	2.3
6	0.8	6×10^{-3}	2.2
7	0.85	7×10^{-3}	2.2
8	0.9	8×10^{-3}	2.1
9	0.95	9×10^{-3}	2.0

The use of this approximation would result in a more accurate value for the pH of a solution with a $[\overset{+}{H}]$ concentration of 5×10^{-3}. The value of 2.3 compares favorably with the value obtained by use of a logarithm table.

If the pH of a solution is known and the $[\overset{+}{H}]$ is desired, the calculation may be carried out as follows.

Examples

If pH = 4.5 and pH = $-\log [\overset{+}{H}]$,

then $\log [\overset{+}{H}] = -$ pH $= -4.5$. This number can be expressed as

$(-5 + 0.5)$ or $0.5 - 5$, and therefore $[\overset{+}{H}]$ would equal antilog $(0.5 - 5)$,

or antilog $0.5 \times$ antilog -5, or 3.16×10^{-5}.

If pH = 2.3, what is the [$\overset{+}{H}$]?

pH = 2.3 = -log [$\overset{+}{H}$]

log [$\overset{+}{H}$] = -2.3 = (-3 + 0.7) = 0.7 - 3

[$\overset{+}{H}$] = antilog (0.7 - 3) = antilog 0.7 × antilog - 3

[$\overset{+}{H}$] = 5.012 × 10^{-3}

EXERCISES

1. A 0.01 N acetic acid solution is 3 per cent ionized. Calculate the [$\overset{+}{H}$] concentration.

2. A 0.1 N HCl solution is 95 per cent ionized. Calculate the [$\overset{+}{H}$] concentration.

3. An acid solution has 1/10,000 g of [$\overset{+}{H}$] per liter. Express the [$\overset{+}{H}$] concentration in terms that would permit you to mentally calculate the pH. What is the pH?

4. Mentally estimate the pH of a solution with a [$\overset{+}{H}$] concentration of 0.0004 (4 × 10^{-4}).

5. A 0.02 N H_3PO_4 solution is 70 per cent ionized. Calculate the [$\overset{+}{H}$] concentration. Mentally estimate the pH and then calculate the actual pH.

6. A biological fluid had a [$\overset{+}{H}$] concentration of 0.0000000312. What is the pH of the fluid?

7. An acid solution had a pH of 3.5. Calculate its [$\overset{+}{H}$] concentration.

6
Buffers

THE *PRACTICAL OBJECTIVES* OF THIS CHAPTER ARE TO OBTAIN
AN UNDERSTANDING OF:

1. The derivation and use of the Henderson-Hasselbalch equation.

2. The calculation of the pK and pH of a buffer solution.

3. The application of the Henderson-Hasselbalch equation in acid-base
   and pCO_2 calculations.

In the last chapter we discussed the dissociation of water and acids and the
calculation of the hydrogen ion concentration and pH. As you doubtless know,
buffer systems consist of a mixture of a weak acid and its salt and are capable of
resisting, or buffering, additions of acids or bases. The ionization constant for a
weak acid, such as acetic acid, is equal to the product of the ionic concentrations
divided by the concentration of the undissociated acid. All concentrations are
usually expressed in moles per liter but may also be expressed in millimoles or
milliequivalents per liter. The ionization constant of a weak acid is usually
designated as K_a, and we may write the equilibrium equation for acetic acid as
follows:

$$HC_2H_3O_2 \rightleftarrows \overset{+}{H} + C_2H_3O_2^-$$

$$K_a = \frac{[\overset{+}{H}] \times [C_2H_3O_2^-]}{[HC_2H_3O_2]}$$

Even though any weak acid and weak base can be used to prepare a buffer
solution, most buffers are composed of a weak acid and weak base that are
conjugates of each other. The acetate buffer, for example, employs acetic acid as
the weak acid and acetate ion as the weak base. The preparation of such a buffer
may involve the direct addition of acetic acid and an acetate salt to water, or the
partial neutralization of an acetic acid solution by a strong base, such as sodium
hydroxide, or the partial neutralization of an acetate salt solution by a strong
acid, such as hydrochloric acid. The ratio of acetic acid to acetate ion in solution
may be chosen to give the desired $[\overset{+}{H}]$ or pH for the buffer solution. If we
rearrange the equilibrium equation of acetic acid:

$$K_a = \frac{[\overset{+}{H}] \times [C_2H_3O_2^-]}{[HC_2H_3O_2]} \quad \text{to} \quad [\overset{+}{H}] = K_a \times \frac{[HC_2H_3O_2]}{[C_2H_3O_2^-]}$$

The $[\overset{+}{H}]$ of the buffer could be calculated from the values for K_a and the concentrations of acid and acetate ion. To convert to the pH and pK notation we could first express the equation in logarithmic form as follows:

$$\log [\overset{+}{H}] = \log K_a + \log \frac{[HC_2H_3O_2]}{[C_2H_3O_2^-]}$$

Since pH and $pK_a = -\log [\overset{+}{H}]$ and $-\log K_a$, the equation could be written as

$$- \log [\overset{+}{H}] = - \log K_a - \log \frac{[HC_2H_3O_2]}{[C_2H_3O_2^-]}$$

by multiplying each term by -1,

$$\text{or as } pH = pK_a - \log \frac{[HC_2H_3O_2]}{[C_2H_3O_2^-]}$$

Finally to retain a positive log function:

$$pH = pK_a + \log \frac{[C_2H_3O_2^-]}{[HC_2H_3O_2]}$$

If we substitute [salt] for $[C_2H_3O_2^-]$ and [acid] for $[HC_2H_3O_2]$, we obtain the **Henderson-Hasselbalch equation,** which is used for the calculation of buffers in general and of acid-base problems involving body fluids in particular.

$$pH = pK + \log \frac{[salt]}{[acid]}$$

The **maximum buffer capacity** of a buffer *in vitro* is obtained when equal concentrations of salt and acid are present. Under these conditions, as, for example, when the acid is half neutralized in a titration, the equation may be expressed as:

$$pH = pK + \log \frac{1}{1} = pK + 0 = pK$$

This represents a practical method of determining **the pK of a buffer.** Values for the pK of acids and bases may also be found in tables in appropriate handbooks.

Examples

The pK_a values for acetic acid and carbonic acid are 4.73 and 6.10, respectively. Calculate the dissociation constant for each acid. Which is the stronger acid?

$$\text{Since } pK_a = - \log K_a, \log K_a = -pK_a$$

For acetic acid

$$\log \ K_a = -4.73 = (-5 + 0.26) = 0.26 - 5$$
$$K_a = \text{antilog } 0.26 \times \text{antilog} - 5$$
$$= 1.8 \times 10^{-5}$$

For carbonic acid

$$pK_a = - \log 6.10$$
$$\log \ K_a = -6.10 = (-7 + 0.9) = 0.9 - 7$$
$$K_a = \text{antilog } 0.9 \times \text{antilog} - 7$$
$$= 7.95 \times 10^{-7}$$

From the K_a values, acetic acid $K_a = 1.8 \times 10^{-5}$ is more completely dissociated and is a stronger acid than carbonic acid, $K_a = 7.9 \times 10^{-7}$.

If 10 ml of 0.05 M acid, when mixed with 10 ml of 0.1 M solution of its sodium salt, gave a solution with a pH of 5.03, what is the pK_a of the acid? The total volume of the final solution is 20 ml; therefore, the final concentration of acid is $10/20 \times 0.05$ M = 0.025 M and the final concentration of the salt is $10/20 \times 0.1$ M = 0.05 M. The fraction:

$$\frac{[\text{salt}]}{[\text{acid}]} = \frac{0.05 \text{ M}}{0.025 \text{ M}} = 2.0$$

and from the Henderson-Hasselbalch equation:

$$pH = pK_a + \log \frac{[\text{salt}]}{[\text{acid}]} \ ; \quad 5.03 = pK_a + \log 2$$

or $5.03 = pK_a + 0.3$ and $pK_a = 5.03 - 0.3 = 4.73$

What amounts (in grams) of sodium acetate and acetic acid are required to prepare 1 liter of 0.1 M buffer with a pH of 5.0? The pK is 4.73. From the Henderson-Hasselbalch equation:

$$pH = pK + \log \frac{[\text{salt}]}{[\text{acid}]} \ ; 5.0 = 4.73 + \log \frac{[\text{salt}]}{[\text{acid}]}$$

Since the total acetate concentration is to be 0.1 M:

$$\text{moles salt/l} + \text{moles acid/l} = 0.1 \text{ moles/l}.$$

From the equation $\log \dfrac{[\text{salt}]}{[\text{acid}]} = 5.0 - 4.73 = 0.27$

$$\dfrac{[\text{salt}]}{[\text{acid}]} = \text{antilog of } 0.27 = 1.862$$

Therefore [salt] = 1.862 [acid].

Since salt + acid = 0.1 moles/l

$$\text{moles salt}/l = 0.1 - \text{moles acid}/l$$

and substituting 1.862 moles acid/l for moles salt/l

$$1.862 \text{ moles acid}/l = 0.1 - \text{moles acid}/l$$

$$\text{or } 2.862 \text{ moles acid}/l = 0.1$$

and moles acid/l $= \dfrac{0.1}{2.862} = 0.0349$ moles acetic acid/l

then moles salt/l = 0.1 − 0.0349 = 0.0651 moles sodium acetate/l.

Weight of acetic acid per liter = 0.0349 × 60 (mol. wt.) = 2.094 g.
Weight of sodium acetate per liter = 0.0651 × 82 (mol. wt.) = 5.345 g.

Therefore, 5.345 g of sodium acetate and 2.094 g of acetic acid when dissolved and diluted to 1 liter will produce a 0.1 M acetate buffer with a pH of 5.0.

Given a buffer solution composed of 10 ml of 0.2 M sodium acetate and 10 ml of 0.2 M acetic acid; what pH change in the solution would result from the addition of 1 ml of 0.2 M HCl? The pK is 4.73. From the Henderson-Hasselbalch equation:

$$pH = pK + \log \dfrac{[\text{salt}]}{[\text{acid}]}$$

The original pH would be: $\quad pH = pK + \log \dfrac{0.1 \text{ M}}{0.1 \text{ M}}$

$$pH = 4.73 + \log \dfrac{0.1}{0.1} = 4.73$$

Since the concentrations of the three solutions are equimolar, we could substitute volumes for concentrations as:

$$pH = 4.73 + \log \frac{10}{10} = 4.73$$

then after the addition of the HCl the equation would be:

$$pH = 4.73 + \log \frac{9}{11} = 4.73 + \log 9 - \log 11$$

$$= 4.73 + 0.954 - 1.041 = 4.64$$

The ratio changes from 10/10 to 9/11 since the HCl would convert 1 ml of the salt to 1 ml of the acid.

Calculate the pH of a bicarbonate buffer that would result from mixing 25 ml of 0.10 M carbonic acid with 25 ml of 0.50 M sodium bicarbonate solution. The pK is 6.10.

Since the total volume is 50 ml, the acid concentration is $\frac{25}{50} \times 0.10$ M = 0.05 M, and the salt concentration is $\frac{25}{50} \times 0.50$ M = 0.25 M.

From the Henderson-Hasselbalch equation

$$pH = pK + \log \frac{[salt]}{[acid]} = 6.10 + \log \frac{0.25 \text{ M}}{0.05 \text{ M}}$$

or pH = 6.10 + log 5 = 6.10 + 0.699 = 6.799.

In the preparation of a phosphate buffer in the biologic range, 6.0 ml of 0.1 M Na_2HPO_4 was mixed with 4.0 ml of O. 1 M KH_2PO_4. The pK is 6.8. What is the pH of the buffer solution?

From the Henderson-Hasselbalch equation

$$pH = pK + \log \frac{[salt]}{[acid]} = 6.8 + \log \frac{6.0 \text{ ml } 0.1 \text{ M}}{4.0 \text{ ml } 0.1 \text{ M}}$$

Since the concentrations of the two solutions are equimolar, we can substitute volumes in the equation, as:

$$pH = 6.8 + \log \frac{6.0}{4.0} = 6.8 + \log 1.5 = 6.8 + 0.176 = 6.976.$$

EXERCISES

A. Calculate the pH of a bicarbonate buffer that is composed of a solution with a final concentration of 0.50 M sodium bicarbonate and 0.05 M carbonic acid. The pK is 6.10.

B. If 16.4 g of sodium acetate and 1.2 g of acetic acid are dissolved and made to volume in a 1 liter volumetric flask, what is the resultant pH of the buffer? The pK is 4.73, the molecular weight of sodium acetate is 82 and the molecular weight of acetic acid is 60.

C. If 20 ml of 0.1 M acid, when mixed with 20 ml of 0.3 M solution of its sodium salt, gave a solution with a pH of 6.58, what is the pK_a of the acid?

D. Given a buffer solution composed of 100 ml of 0.1 M sodium acetate and 100 ml of 0.1 M acetic acid, what pH change would result from the addition of 5.0 ml of 0.1 M HCl. The pK_a is 4.73. (Hint: the concentrations are all 0.1 M.)

6.1 ACID-BASE BUFFER CALCULATIONS

In addition to hemoglobin, the $\dfrac{HCO_3^-}{H_2CO_3}$ buffer system is primarily responsible for the **transport of CO_2 and the control of blood pH**. The Henderson-Hasselbalch equation representing this important blood buffer was originally written as:

$$pH = pK_a + \log \frac{[HCO_3^-]}{[H_2CO_3]}$$

The pK_a for the buffer is 6.1 and normal values for $[HCO_3^-]$ and $[H_2CO_3]$ average 27 and 1.35 mM/l, respectively. Under normal conditions the pH of the blood averages 7.4; substituting these values in the equation:

$$7.4 = 6.1 + \log \frac{27 \ mM/l}{1.35 \ mM/l}$$

or

$$7.4 = 6.1 + \log 20 = 6.1 + 1.3 = 7.4$$

The normal ratio of bicarbonate to carbonic acid of 20:1 is maintained by the buffer with the assistance of the lungs and the kidneys. Changes in this ratio are seen in respiratory and metabolic acid-base imbalances. For example, an initial change in bicarbonate concentration to one half the normal value without any change in carbonic acid concentration occurred in a rapidly developing metabolic acidosis. What change would occur in the blood pH?

From the Henderson-Hasselbalch equation:

$$pH = pK + \log \frac{[HCO_3^-]}{[H_2CO_3]}$$

$$= 6.1 + \log \frac{13.5 \text{ mM/l}}{1.35 \text{ mM/l}}$$

$$= 6.1 + \log 10 = 6.1 + 1.0 = 7.1$$

A major problem that concerns the use of the Henderson-Hasselbalch equation in the above form is the fact that free carbonic acid is not readily measured. It is, however, in equilibrium with and proportional to the dissolved CO_2, which is also directly proportional to **the partial pressure of CO_2 (pCO_2)**. These statements may be illustrated as follows:

$$H_2CO_3 \rightleftarrows CO_2 + H_2O \rightleftarrows \alpha p CO_2 \text{ (dissolved } CO_2) \rightleftarrows p CO_2$$

If we substitute $\alpha p CO_2$ for $[H_2CO_3]$

$$pH = pK + \log \frac{[HCO_3^-]}{\alpha p CO_2}$$

Since the total CO_2 of the blood = $[HCO_3^-] + [H_2CO_3]$, the $[HCO_3^-]$ = total $CO_2 - [H_2CO_3]$ or total $CO_2 - \alpha p CO_2$. Substituting again:

$$pH = pK + \log \left[\frac{\text{Total } CO_2 - \alpha p CO_2}{\alpha p CO_2} \right]$$

The proportionality constant, α, is derived from the solubility coefficient of CO_2 (ml of CO_2 dissolved per ml of solvent = 0.5311 at 37°C) by the following equation:

$$mM/l \ CO_2 = \frac{1000 \text{ ml/l} \times 0.5311 \times pCO_2}{760 \text{ mm Hg} \times 22.26 \text{ ml/mM}} = 0.0314 \ pCO_2$$

The approximate proportionality constant for CO_2 = 0.03, so using known values:

$$pH = 6.1 + \log \left[\frac{\text{Total } CO_2 - 0.03 \ p CO_2}{0.03 \ p CO_2} \right]$$

When total CO_2 is expressed in mM/l and pCO_2 as mm Hg, the expression for pCO_2 becomes:

$$pCO_2 \text{ (mm Hg)} = \frac{\text{Total } CO_2 \text{ mM/l}}{0.03 \text{ [antilog (pH} - 6.1) + 1]}$$

Examples:

What is the pCO_2 of plasma with total CO_2 of 28 mM/l and a pH of 7.50?

From the equation:

$$pCO_2 = \frac{\text{Total } CO_2}{0.03 \text{ [antilog (pH} - 6.1) + 1]}$$

$$= \frac{28}{0.03 \text{ [antilog (7.5} - 6.1) + 1]}$$

$$= \frac{28}{0.03 \text{ [antilog (1.4)} + 1]} = \frac{28}{0.03 \text{ [25.1} + 1]}$$

$$= \frac{28}{0.03 \text{ [26.1]}} = \frac{28}{0.783} = 35.8$$

Therefore the pCO_2 = 35.8 mm Hg

Calculate the pH of plasma that has a total CO_2 of 26.1 mM/l and a pCO_2 of 40.5 mm Hg.

From the Henderson-Hasselbalch equation,

$$pH = pK + \log \frac{[HCO_3^-]}{[H_2CO_3]}$$

First calculate the $[H_2CO_3]$ and the $[HCO_3^-]$.

$$[H_2CO_3] = \alpha pCO_2 = 0.03 \times 40.5 = 1.22 \text{ mM/l}$$

$$[HCO_3^-] = \text{total } CO_2 - [H_2CO_3] = 26.1 - 1.22 = 24.88 \text{ mM/l}$$

Then $pH = 6.1 + \log \dfrac{24.88}{1.22} = 6.1 + \log 20.4 = 6.1 + 1.310 = 7.410$

Since the equation just employed is rather complex for routine calculations in the laboratory, several schemes have been devised to simplify the problem. These include **nomograms** (Appendix), which illustrate the relationships existing in the Henderson-Hasselbalch equation which permit the determination of pCO_2 graphically if the total CO_2 and the pH are known. In addition **special slide rules** have been devised to facilitate calculations involving the equation. Another method requires a total CO_2 content determination of anaerobically separated plasma plus a determination of whole blood or "true" plasma pH at $38°C$. An equation is then set up as follows:

$$pCO_2 \text{ (mm Hg)} = \frac{\text{Total } CO_2 \text{ mM/l}}{F}$$

where F is a factor that corresponds to the denominator of the earlier equation 0.03 [antilog (pH − 6.1) + 1] and is calculated for each pH value at a temperature of $38°C$. A portion of an available table of factor F versus pH at $38°C$ is reproduced to illustrate the method.

TABLE 6.1 FACTORS FOR pCO_2 CALCULATIONS

pH	Factor F	pH	Factor F	pH	Factor F
7.10	0.331	7.26	0.465	7.42	0.659
7.12	0.345	7.28	0.486	7.44	0.689
7.14	0.360	7.30	0.507	7.46	0.720
7.16	0.376	7.32	0.530	7.48	0.752
7.18	0.392	7.34	0.553	7.50	0.786
7.20	0.409	7.36	0.578	7.52	0.822
7.22	0.427	7.38	0.604	7.54	0.859
7.24	0.445	7.40	0.631	7.56	0.898

As a sample calculation we may determine the pCO_2 of plasma with a total CO_2 of 28 mM/l and a pH of 7.50, as used in the last example.

From the equation:

$$pCO_2 = \frac{\text{Total } CO_2}{F}$$

F from the table = 0.786; therefore,

$$pCO_2 = \frac{28}{0.786} = 35.6 \text{ mm Hg}$$

This value for pCO_2 compares favorably with the 35.8 mm Hg obtained with the full equation.

ADDITIONAL EXERCISES

1. A patient with the symptoms of metabolic acidosis had plasma values of 20 mM/l and 1.5 mM/l for bicarbonate and carbonic acid concentrations, respectively. What was the pH of the plasma?

2. Calculate the pCO_2 of a patient's plasma if the pH is 7.33 and the total CO_2 is 24 mM/l.

3. Using the table of factors, calculate the pCO_2 if the total CO_2 of the plasma is 37 mM/l and the pH is 7.56.

4. If a patient's plasma has a pH of 7.10 and a pCO_2 of 78 mm Hg, calculate the total CO_2 content in mM/l, using the table of factors.

5. What is the pH of the plasma of a patient whose bicarbonate and carbonic acid concentrations are 35 mM/l and 1.25 mM/l, respectively?

6. What value for plasma bicarbonate would be obtained on analysis of a serum specimen with the following characteristics: pH 7.20 and carbonic acid 2.0 mM/l?

7. Using the table of factors, calculate the total CO_2 of a plasma specimen with a pH of 7.38 and a pCO_2 of 42 mm Hg.

8. Calculate the pCO_2 of a patient's plasma if the pH is 7.48 and the total CO_2 is 27.5 mM/l?

7
Renal Clearance
Test Calculations

> THE *PRACTICAL OBJECTIVES* OF THIS CHAPTER ARE TO OBTAIN
> AN UNDERSTANDING OF:
>
> 1. The concept of renal clearance and its application to the calculation of
>   clearance values.
>
> 2. The importance of body surface correction in accurate clearance
>   calculations.

7.1 UREA CLEARANCE TEST

One of the first generally accepted tests of the overall function of the kidney
was the urea clearance test. Urea undergoes both glomerular filtration and
tubular reabsorption, and its clearance from the plasma is expressed as the
milliliters of plasma that contain the amount of urea excreted by the kidneys
each minute. Obviously the plasma is not completely cleared of urea because of
the constant tubular reabsorption, but the common expression for clearance is
the **milliliters of plasma cleared per minute.** Since the rate of urea reabsorption
depends on the rate of reabsorption of water, we take this fact into considera-
tion by using either the formula for **maximum clearance** (urine excretion rate
2.0 ml/min or more) or that for **standard clearance** (urine excretion rate up to
2.0 ml/min)

7.2 MAXIMUM CLEARANCE

Urea clearance tests are more significant when the urine excretion rate is 2.0
ml/min or more. Tubular reabsorption of urea has less influence on the test at
this rate. Maximum clearance is calculated as follows:

$$C_{max} = \frac{U \times V}{S}$$

where C_{max} is expressed in ml/min; the concentration of urea in the urine (U)
and serum (S) are both expressed in mg/100 ml, and V, the volume of urine, is

expressed in ml/min. **The average normal maximum clearance is 75 ml/min**, and because there is also a standard urea clearance calculation, the clearances are often reported in per cent of the normal clearance.

Example

A patient's serum urea was 12 mg/dl, the urine urea was 222 mg/dl and the total urine volume for a 2 hour test period was 360 ml. The rate of urine excretion would be

$$\frac{360 \text{ ml}}{120 \text{ min}} = 3 \text{ ml/min}$$

Using the above equation:

$$C_{max} = \frac{U \times V}{S} = \frac{222 \times 3}{12} = \frac{666}{12} = 55.5 \text{ ml/min}$$

Therefore C_{max} = 55.5 ml/min or $\frac{55.5}{75}$ = 74 per cent of normal

7.3 STANDARD CLEARANCE

When the urine excretion rate is less than 2.0 ml/min, the normal urea clearance values drop below 75 ml/min. Since this decrease in clearance rate is approximately proportional to the square root of the urine excretion rate, the standard urea clearance is calculated as follows:

$$C_{std} = \frac{U \times \sqrt{V}}{S}$$

The average normal standard urea clearance is 54 ml/min.

Example

A patient's serum urea was 24 mg/dl, the urine urea 600 mg/dl and the total urine volume for a 2 hour test period was 180 ml. The rate of urine excretion would be

$$\frac{180}{120} = 1.5 \text{ ml/min}$$

Using the above equation:

$$C_{std} = \frac{U \times \sqrt{V}}{S} = \frac{600 \times \sqrt{1.5}}{24} = \frac{600 \times 1.23}{24} = \frac{735}{24} = 30.6 \text{ ml/min}$$

Therefore C_{std} = 30.6 ml/min or $\frac{30.6}{54}$ = 56.7 per cent of normal.

7.4 CREATININE CLEARANCE

In many laboratories the creatinine clearance test has replaced the urea clearance test as a measure of kidney function. Creatinine is predominantly excreted by glomerular filtration and therefore serves as an indicator of glomerular filtration rate. Since tubular reabsorption is minimal, we need not be concerned about maximum or standard clearances or per cent of normal clearance values. The calculation employs the simple relationship:

$$C = \frac{U \times V}{S}$$

Example

A patient's serum creatinine was 1.1 mg/dl, the urine creatinine 45 mg/dl and the urine volume for a 4 hour test period was 550 ml. The rate of urine excretion would be

$$\frac{550}{240} = 2.3 \text{ ml/min}$$

Using the above equation:

$$C = \frac{U \times V}{S} = \frac{45 \times 2.3}{1.1} = 94.2 \text{ ml/min}$$

Therefore the creatinine clearance is 94.2 ml/min, which may be compared to an average normal glomerular filtration rate of 125 ml/min for men and 115 ml/min for women.

To obtain meaningful comparisons of renal clearance rates for patients of various sizes and weights **the results must often be corrected for body surface.**

This correction is obviously important in pediatrics. In adults the average body surface is taken as 1.73 square meters, and clearance test rates in both adults and children are corrected by the following formula:

$$C \times \frac{1.73}{A} = \text{ml/min corrected for body surface}$$

where A is the body surface of the patient in square meters. **Tables and nomograms** (see Appendix) are available that yield body surface values in square meters when the patient's weight is expressed in kilograms (or pounds) and their height in centimeters (or feet and inches). If these aids are not available, the body surface may be calculated by a complex formula:

$$\text{Log } A = 0.425 \log W + 0.725 \log H - 2.144$$

where A is the body surface in square meters, W is the weight in kilograms and H is the height in centimeters.

Example

A patient weighs 120 pounds and is 5 feet 2 inches in height. The weight in kilograms = 120/2.2 = 54.5 kg and the height in centimeters = 62 inches × 2.54 cm/in = 157.6 cm.

From the above equation:

$$\text{Log } A = 0.425 \log W + 0.725 \log H - 2.144$$

$$= 0.425 \times \log 54.5 + 0.725 \times \log 157.6 - 2.144$$

$$= 0.425 \times 1.747 + 0.725 \times 2.198 - 2.144$$

$$= 0.744 + 1.592 - 2.144$$

$$= 2.336 - 2.144$$

$$= 0.192$$

$$A = \text{antilog } 0.192 = 1.555 \text{ square meters}$$

The results of a creatinine clearance test on this patient were as follows: serum creatinine 1.2 mg/dl, urine creatinine 48 mg/dl and urine volume for a 4 hour test period was 500 ml. Calculate the creatinine clearance corrected for body surface.

From the equation:

$$C = \frac{U \times V}{S} = \frac{48 \times 2.08}{1.2} = 99.8 \text{ ml/min}$$

From the equation:

$$C \times \frac{1.73}{A} = \text{ml/min corrected for body surface}$$

$$99.8 \times \frac{1.73}{1.555} = 110.0 \text{ ml/min}$$

EXERCISES

1. Calculate the urea clearance and per cent of normal from the following data. Serum urea 15 mg/dl, urine urea 325 mg/dl and urine volume for a 2 hour test period was 300 ml.

2. A patient with glomerulonephritis excreted 120 ml of urine in a 2 hour test period. The urine contained 750 mg of urea per 100 ml and the serum 50 mg/dl. Calculate the clearance and per cent normal for this patient.

3. A patient's serum creatinine was 1.4 mg/dl, the urine creatinine 50 mg/dl and the urine volume for a 4 hour test period was 720 ml. Calculate the creatinine clearance.

4. A child weighed 25 pounds and was 2 feet tall. Calculate the body surface in square meters.

5. A child 4 feet 4 inches tall weighed 60 pounds. A creatinine clearance was run with a result of 95 ml/min (uncorrected). Correct the clearance for the child's body surface.

6. From the following data, calculate the creatinine clearance of the patient corrected for body surface. Serum creatinine was 0.9 mg/dl, urine creatinine 48 mg/dl, urine volume 2.2 ml/min, body weight 110 pounds and height 5 feet.

7. A large patient who was 6 feet 4 inches tall and weighed 240 pounds excreted 360 ml of urine in a 2 hour urea clearance test. The serum urea concentration was 12 mg/dl, and the urine urea was 400 mg/dl. Calculate the urea clearance corrected for body surface.

8
Spectrophotometric Calculations

THE *PRACTICAL OBJECTIVES* OF THIS CHAPTER ARE TO OBTAIN AN UNDERSTANDING OF:

1. The use of molar extinction coefficient calculations in the laboratory.

2. The application of Beer's law in the calculation of the concentration of constituents in biologic fluids.

The majority of the determinations carried out in the clinical chemistry laboratory depend on measurements made with a spectrophotometer. These instruments measure the amount of light absorbed by a particular substance in solution or a color produced by a colored derivative of that substance in the visible range, the near ultraviolet and ultraviolet range and in the infrared range. **Calculations involving spectrophotometric data are based on Beer's law.** Beer's law states that the concentration of a substance is directly proportional to the amount of light absorbed or inversely proportional to the logarithm of the transmitted light. The mathematical equation representing Beer's law is as follows:

$$A = abc = \log \frac{100}{\% \, T} = 2 - \log \% \, T$$

where A = absorbance, a = absorptivity, b = light path of solution in centimeters, c = concentration of the substance in solution and $\% \, T$ = per cent transmittance.

Although some spectrophotometers have only a $\% \, T$ scale, the majority have both A and $\% \, T$ scales, and the modern trend is toward linear A scales. In the above equation when the concentration units are moles per liter, a is called the molar absorptivity or the **molar extinction coefficient** and is designated ϵ. In spectrophotometry ϵ is defined as the absorbance (optical density) of a one molar solution of 1 cm thickness. From the equation:

$$A = abc = \epsilon bc$$

81

when b = 1 cm and c = 1 molar, A = ϵ.

The measurement of the molar extinction coefficient is often used to determine the purity of a compound with a known molecular weight. An example is the determination of the purity of bilirubin in clinical laboratories. A joint commission of pathologists and clinical chemists recommended that bilirubin preparations having an ϵ between 59,100 and 62,300 at a wavelength of 453 nm in chloroform at 25°C were suitable for standards.

Examples

A bilirubin solution in chloroform at 25°C measured at a wavelength of 453 nm in a 1 cm light path cuvette gave an absorbance of 0.528. The concentration of the solution was 5 mg bilirubin per liter. Calculate the molar extinction coefficient.

From the equation A = ϵbc or $\epsilon = \dfrac{A}{bc}$

$$c = 5 \text{ mg/l (mol. wt. = 572)}$$

$$\text{c in moles/l} = \frac{0.005 \text{ g/l}}{572 \text{ g/l}} = 0.00000873 \text{ or } 8.73 \times 10^{-6} \text{ M}$$

$$\text{Then } \epsilon = \frac{A}{1 \times 8.73 \times 10^{-6} \text{ M}} = \frac{0.528}{8.73 \times 10^{-6} \text{ M}} = \frac{5.28 \times 10^{-1}}{8.73 \times 10^{-6}}$$

$$= 0.605 \times 10^{-1 \, - \, (-6)} = 0.605 \times 10^{5} = 60,500$$

A purified bilirubin preparation was found to have an extinction coefficient of 61,500 under the conditions described above. What concentration of this bilirubin expressed in mg/l would produce an absorbance of 0.850 at 453 nm in a 1 cm light path cuvette at 25°C?

From the equation A = ϵbc, $c = \dfrac{A}{\epsilon b}$

$$c = \frac{0.850}{61,500 \times 1} = \frac{8.50 \times 10^{-1}}{6.15 \times 10^{4}} = 1.38 \times 10^{-1 \, - \, (4)}$$

$$= 1.38 \times 10^{-5}$$

Therefore c = 1.38×10^{-5} M = $\dfrac{X \text{ g/l}}{572 \text{ g/l}}$ or X = $1.38 \times 10^{-5} \times 572$ or X = $1.38 \times 10^{-5} \times 5.72 \times 10^{-2} = 7.9 \times 10^{-3}$ g/l = 7.9 mg/l.

EXERCISES

A. Calculate the molar extinction coefficient of a compound in a solution containing 0.1 mM per liter that produced an absorbance of 0.425 at 420 nm in a 1 cm light path cuvette.

B. What absorbance value would result from reading a bilirubin solution, 1.0 mg/dl, ϵ = 62,000 in a 1 cm light path cuvette at 453 nm at 25°C?

A more common type of calculation that is employed in spectrophotometric measurements involves the determination of the concentration of a known constituent in a biological fluid. From Beer's law the absorbance A of a solution of concentration C_1 is directly proportional to the absorbance A_2 of the same solution at a different concentration, C_2, or

$$\frac{A_1}{A_2} = \frac{C_1}{C_2}$$

$$\text{therefore } C_1 = \frac{A_1}{A_2} \times C_2$$

If solution 2 is a standard solution of known concentration and solution 1 a biological fluid of unknown concentration, then:

$$C_u = \frac{A_u}{A_s} \times C_s \text{ or in terms of } \% \text{ T}$$

$$C_u = \frac{2 - \log \% T_u}{2 - \log \% T_s} \times C_s$$

Example

An example of a simple problem would be the calculation of the concentration of a constituent in urine when 1 ml of urine and 1 ml of a standard solution of the constituent containing 0.4 mg were treated by a reaction that produced an absorbance of 0.325 for the standard solution and 0.350 for the urine.

From the equation:

$$C_u = \frac{A_u}{A_s} \times C_s$$

$$C_u = \frac{0.350}{0.325} \times 0.4 \text{ mg} = 0.431 \text{ mg/ml of urine}$$

The same problem using % T values instead of absorbance would result in readings of 47.3% T for the standard solution and 44.6% T for the urine.

From the equation:

$$C_u = \frac{2 - \log \% T_u}{2 - \log \% T_s} \times C_s$$

$$2 - \log \% T_u = 2 - \log 44.6 = 2 - 1.65 = 0.35$$

$$2 - \log \% T_s = 2 - \log 47.3 = 2 - 1.675 = 0.325$$

$$C_u = \frac{0.350}{0.325} \times 0.4 \text{ mg} = 0.431 \text{ mg/ml urine}$$

When a dilution of serum, urine or a protein-free filtrate is used in a spectrophotometric determination or when the amount of a constituent in a definite volume of a biological fluid is desired, the calculation is more involved.

Examples

A patient excreted 1500 ml of urine in 24 hours. A 1 ml aliquot of the urine and 1 ml of a standard creatinine solution containing 0.8 mg were treated with an alkaline picrate solution with a resulting absorbance of 0.285 for the standard and 0.275 for the urine when read at 530 nm. Calculate the 24 h excretion of creatinine.

From the equation:

$$C_u = \frac{A_u}{A_s} \times C_s \; ; C_u = \frac{0.275}{0.285} \times 0.8 \text{ mg} = 0.772 \text{ mg/ml}$$

Total volume: 1500 ml $\times$ 0.772 mg/ml = 1158 mg/24 h

A 1 ml aliquot of a 1:10 protein-free filtrate from serum and 0.2 ml of a standard phosphate solution containing 0.003 mg P diluted to a volume of 1 ml with water were treated with an aminonaphtholsulfonic acid solution to produce a blue color that was diluted to 25 ml in each determination; the absorbances were read at 660 nm. The reading of the standard solution was 0.410 and of the protein-free filtrate 0.450. Calculate the phosphate concentration in mg/dl in the serum.

From the equation:

$$C_u = \frac{A_u}{A_s} \times C_s \; ; C_u = \frac{0.450}{0.410} \times 0.003 \text{ mg} = 0.00329 \text{ mg}$$

$$C_u = 0.00329 \text{ mg in } \frac{1}{10} \text{ ml serum} = 10 \times 0.00329 = 0.0329 \text{ mg/ml}$$

$$\text{or } 100 \times 0.0329 \text{ mg} = 3.29 \text{ mg/dl P in serum}$$

ADDITIONAL EXERCISES

1. A vitamin D solution in alcohol at 25°C measured at a wavelength of 264 nm in a 1 cm light path cuvette gave an absorbance of 0.218. The concentration of the solution was 5 mg/l and the molecular weight is 397. Calculate the molar extinction coefficient.

2. Using the molar extinction coefficient found in problem 1 for vitamin D, calculate the absorbance at 264 nm in a 1 cm light path cuvette at 25°C produced by a solution whose concentration was 12.5 mg/l.

3. A 1 ml aliquot of urine and 1 ml of a standard creatinine solution containing 0.4 mg were treated with an alkaline picrate solution with a resulting absorbance of 0.582 for the standard and 0.560 for the urine when read at 530 nm. Calculate the creatinine excretion in mg/dl.

4. To a 4 ml aliquot of a 1:10 protein free filtrate from serum and 4 ml of a standard creatinine solution containing 0.00115 mg/ml were added 2 ml of an alkaline picrate solution. After 15 minutes the absorbance readings at 530 nm were as follows: protein free filtrate aliquot 0.365, standard 0.350. What was the creatinine concentration of the serum in mg/dl?

5. A series of standard phosphate solutions was treated with an amino-naphtholsulfonic acid solution to produce a blue color that was diluted to 25 ml in each determination and the absorbances were read at 660 nm.

Phosphate equiv. to mg/dl	Absorbance
0	0.003
1.0	0.150
2.0	0.295
3.0	0.459
4.0	0.595
5.0	0.725

Construct the standard curve plotting the concentration (abscissa) against the absorbance (ordinate). Does the curve follow Beer's law throughout the entire range of concentrations? Explain.

6. From the standard curve prepared in Problem 5, determine the serum phosphate concentrations of the following specimens that were treated the same as the standards.

Absorbance readings
a. 0.625
b. 0.505
c. 0.495
d. 0.640

7. A flame emission spectrophotometer set up for the determination of serum sodium gave readings of 19, 40, 59, 81 and 99 on a linear scale when standards containing 110, 120, 130, 140 and 150 mEq/l of sodium respectively were aspirated in the flame. What would be the sodium concentration of the following serum samples that were treated in the same fashion as the standards?

Meter readings
a. 51
b. 83
c. 69
d. 72

Radiologic Calculations

THE *PRACTICAL OBJECTIVES* OF THIS CHAPTER ARE TO OBTAIN
AN UNDERSTANDING OF:

1. The concepts of radioactive decay, the decay constant, the half-life, and methods of calculation.

2. The similarity between calculations of radioactive decay and radiation protection, and the concepts of the linear absorption coefficient and the half-value layer.

3. The differences between the physical, biologic, and the effective half-life of an isotope.

4. The use of specific activity in the calculations of volume and concentration changes in radioactive solutions.

In radiation measurement and protection common calculations involve the determination of radioactive decay of an element with time, the half-life of a radioactive element, the protection afforded by a sheet of absorbing material of a certain thickness, and the half-value layer or thickness of material that will reduce the radioactivity to one half of its original activity. In biologic systems it is also of value to compare and to calculate the radioisotope half-life, the biologic half-life, and the effective half-life. The specific activity of an isotope and its use in calculating concentrations of radioactive solutions may also be important. Quality control parameters useful in measuring radioactivity, such as the chi-square test and quality control curves of the disintegrations per second or per minute, are included in Chapter 11.

9.1 RADIOACTIVE DECAY

When a radioactive nucleus changes to another nucleus, this change is called disintegration or decay. The **rate of decay** is expressed in terms of disintegrations per unit of time. The **curie**, Ci, is defined as a unit of radioactivity with 3.7×10^{10} disintegrations per second, or 2.2×10^{12} disintegrations per minute. A **millicurie**, mCi, would yield 3.7×10^{7} and a **microcurie**, μCi, 3.7×10^{4} disintegrations per second respectively.

Since the rate of decay of a given isotope is constant, a common measure of the decay is called the **physical half-life** ($T_{1/2}$ or T_p) or radioactive half-life of the isotope. This half-life is defined as the length of time required for one half of the original number of atoms in a given radioactive sample to disintegrate. In the decay process, the fraction of the remaining number of atoms which decay per unit of time is called the **decay constant.** λ. To determine the decrease in radioactivity with time, a plot of the number of atoms or counts versus time on semilogarithmic paper (see p. 110) may be used. A number of half-lives may be represented on the time scale, and within the limits of the graph the decrease in radioactivity can be quantitated. The classical equation representing the decay of radioactive materials is as follows:

$$N = N_o e^{-\lambda t} \quad \text{or} \quad I = I_o e^{-\lambda t}$$

where N and I are the number of atoms or the strength of radioactivity present after a period of time, t; N_0 and I_0 are the number of atoms or the strength of radioactivity originally present; e is the base of natural logarithms, 2.718; λ is the decay constant of the particular radioisotope; and t is the time elapsed. This equation may also be expressed as:

$$\frac{I_o}{I} = e^{\lambda t}$$

Referring to tables of natural logarithms, the calculation of radioactive decay is relatively simple. For example, radon has a decay constant of 2.097×10^{-6}/s. If the initial strength of a radon seed is 10 millicuries, its strength three days later may be calculated.

$$\text{From} \frac{I_o}{I} = e^{\lambda t} \text{ we have } \frac{10}{I} = e^{2.097 \times 10^{-6} \times 3 \times 24 \times 60 \times 60}$$

$$\text{or} \frac{10}{1} = e^{0.5435} \text{ and } e^{0.5435} = 1.722 \text{ and } 10 = 1.722 \text{ I}$$

$$\text{or } I = \frac{10}{1.722} = 5.81 \text{ millicuries.}$$

Since natural logarithm tables of values of e^x are not always available and logarithms to the base 10 were covered in Chapter 2, the classical equation is commonly expressed as:

$$\log \frac{I_o}{I} = 0.4343 \, \lambda t \quad \text{or} \quad \log \frac{N_o}{N} = 0.4343 \, \lambda t$$

Examples

Given a source of ^{45}Ca which has a decay constant of 4.26×10^{-3}/day, calculate the per cent of the original activity remaining after 80 days. Substituting in the equation

$$\log \frac{I_0}{I} = 0.4343 \times 4.26 \times 10^{-3} \times 80 = 0.148$$

Let $I_0 = 100\%$; then $\log \frac{100}{I} = 0.148$, or $\log 100 - \log I = 0.148$

and $\log I = \log 100 - 0.148 = 2.000 - 0.148 = 1.852$, or $I = 71.1\%$

A sample of ^{197}Hg has an original activity of 200 μCi. If ^{197}Hg has a decay constant of 0.0107/hour, what will the activity of the sample be after one day?

$$\log \frac{I_0}{I} = 0.4343 \lambda t \quad \text{or} \quad \log \frac{200}{I} = 0.4343 \times 0.0107 \times 24 \text{ h} = 0.1115$$

$$\log \frac{200}{I} = 0.1115 \quad \text{or} \quad \log 200 - \log I = 0.1115$$

and $\log I = \log 200 - 0.1115 = 2.3010 - 0.1115 = 2.1895$,

or $I = 154.6 \mu$Ci.

EXERCISES

A. ^{59}Fe has a decay constant of 0.015/day. What per cent of initial activity will remain after one week?

B. ^{125}I has a decay constant of 0.01155/day. If the original activity of a sample of ^{125}I is 5 mCi, what will be its activity in 4 weeks?

Radioactive decay is often based on the **half-life**, $t_{1/2}$, of a radioactive element. Mathematically it can be proven that

$$t_{1/2} = \frac{0.693}{\lambda} \quad \text{or that} \quad \lambda = \frac{0.693}{t_{1/2}}$$

and therefore

$$\log\frac{I_o}{I} = 0.4343 \times \frac{0.693}{t_{1/2}} \times t$$

If the half-life of a radioactive isotope is known, the decay constant may be calculated or the extent of radioactive decay may be calculated from the last equation.

Examples

From Exercise B, ^{125}I has a decay constant of 0.01155/day. What is the half-life of ^{125}I in days? In seconds?

From the equation $t_{1/2} = \frac{0.693}{\lambda} = \frac{0.693}{0.01155} = 60$ days;

then $60 \times 24 \times 60 \times 60 = 5.184 \times 10^6$ s.

^{131}I has a half-life of 8.1 days. What percentage of a sample of ^{131}I will remain after one week?

From $\log\frac{I_o}{I} = 0.4343 \times \frac{0.693}{t_{1/2}} \times t = 0.4343 \times \frac{0.693}{8.1} \times 7 = 0.2601,$

let $I_o = 100\%$; then $\log\frac{100}{I} = 0.2601$, or $\log 100 - \log I = 0.2601$,

and $\log I = \log 100 - 0.2601 = 2.000 - 0.2601 = 1.7399$,

or $I = 54.94\%$

EXERCISES

C. The half-life of ^{57}Co is 270 days. If the source has an original activity of 10 mCi, what will its activity be after 100 days?

D. ^{32}P has a decay constant of 0.0485/day. What is its half-life in days? If a sample has an initial activity of 300 μCi, how much will be left after 3 weeks?

E. The half-life of ^{15}O is 2.069 minutes. Calculate the decay constant per minute and activity remaining after 80 seconds if the original activity is 20 mCi.

9.2 RADIATION PROTECTION

Fortunately, for ease in calculations, the protection from radioactivity by a sheet of absorbing material involves a simple modification of the equations used to determine radioactive decay and half-life. The classical equation would be expressed as:

$$I = I_0 e^{-\mu d} \quad \text{or} \quad N = N_0 e^{-\mu d}$$

where I_0 and I or N_0 and N are the same as these expressions in the equations in Section 9.1; e is 2.718, the base of natural logarithms; μ is the **linear absorption coefficient** of the sheet of absorbing material; and d is the thickness of the sheet, usually expressed in centimeters. Utilizing logarithms to the base 10, the above equation becomes

$$\log \frac{I_0}{I} = 0.4343 \, \mu d$$

and the **half-value layer,** representing the thickness of a sheet of material which will reduce the intensity of the transmitted radiation to one half, is expressed as

$$d_{1/2} = \frac{0.693}{\mu} \quad \text{or} \quad \mu = \frac{0.693}{d_{1/2}}$$

and therefore

$$\log \frac{I_0}{I} = 0.4343 \times \frac{0.693}{d_{1/2}} \times d$$

Examples

A sheet of absorbing material has a linear absorption coefficient of 0.220/cm for a 100 kev gamma ray source. What per cent of the initial intensity of gamma rays will penetrate 2.3 cm of this material?

From $\log \frac{I_O}{I} = 0.4343\ \mu d = 0.4343 \times 0.220 \times 2.3 = 0.2198$.

Let $\log I_O = 100\%$; then $\log \frac{100}{I} = 0.2198$, or $\log 100 - \log I = 0.2198$,

and $\log I = \log 100 - 0.2198 = 2.000 - 0.2198 = 1.7802$,

or $I = 60.3\%$.

The half-value layer for lead is approximately 0.385 mm for a beam of positrons. What is the linear absorption coefficient for lead in this situation, and what percentage of a beam of positrons will penetrate 0.2 cm of lead?

From $\mu = \dfrac{0.693}{d_{1/2}} = \dfrac{0.693}{0.0385}$ cm $= 18/\text{cm}$.

From $\log \frac{I_O}{I} = 0.4343 \times \dfrac{0.693}{d_{1/2}} \times d = 0.4343 \times \dfrac{0.693}{0.0385} \times 0.2 = 1.563$.

Let $I_O = 100\%$; then $\log \frac{100}{I} = 1.563$ or $\log 100 - \log I = 1.563$,

and $\log I = \log 100 - 1.563 = 2.000 - 1.563 = 0.437$,

or $I = 2.74\%$

If the radiation intensity before shielding is 200 millirads/hour and the linear absorption coefficient of the shielding material is 0.50/cm, what intensity of radiation will penetrate 1.5 cm of the material?

From $\log \frac{I_O}{I} = 0.4343\ \mu d = \log \frac{200}{I} = 0.4343 \times 0.50 \times 1.5$

$\log \frac{200}{I} = 0.3257$ or $\log 200 - \log I = 0.3257$

and $\log I = \log 200 - 0.3257 = 2.3010 - 0.3257 = 1.9753$,

or $\log I = 94.5$ mr/h.

EXERCISES

A. Tissue has a linear absorption coefficient of approximately 0.45/cm for the 27 kev x-rays of ^{125}I. What per cent of these x-rays will pass through 3 cm of tissue?

B. Lead has a linear absorption coefficient of approximately 25/cm for the 140 kev gamma rays of ^{99}Tc. Calculate the half-value layer for lead under these conditions and the per cent of these gamma rays that will pass through a sheet of lead 0.5 mm thick.

C. The half-value layer for tissue is approximately 7.5 cm for a beam of positrons. What per cent of the beam will penetrate 12.5 cm of tissue?

D. If the half-value layer of lead for the radiation source employed is 0.325 mm and the initial radiation intensity is 100 mr/h, what intensity of radiation will penetrate a sheet of lead 0.7 mm thick?

9.3 BIOLOGIC AND EFFECTIVE HALF-LIFE

A radioactive isotope in an inorganic or organic compound when administered to a patient is eliminated from the body at a rate that is proportional to the biologic half-life of that compound. The **biologic half-life** (T_b) is obviously important in predicting radiation damage to the body from internal emitting radionuclides. A radioisotope that is rapidly turned over or eliminated from the body will have a short T_b regardless of the length of its **physical half-life**. Since both the biologic and physical half-lives of a radioisotope are involved in estimating the amount of radiation absorbed by body tissue, a more practical term is used to express the relationship between the two half-lives. This is called the **effective half-life**, and is defined as the time required for the radiation of a given isotope to diminish by 50 per cent as a result of both radioactive decay and biologic elimination.

The effective half-live is usually determined experimentally by administering a dose of a compound containing a radioisotope and measuring the uptake of the isotope by the body by daily counting procedures until the activity reaches 50 per cent of the initial dose. Simple equations for the calculation of the biologic half-life when both the physical half-life (T_p) and effective half-life (T_e) are known, and for calculation of the effective half-life when both the physical and biologic half-lives are known, are as follows:

$$T_b = \frac{T_p \times T_e}{T_p - T_e} \quad \text{and} \quad T_e = \frac{T_p \times T_b}{T_p + T_b}$$

Examples

In an experiment on the ^{131}I uptake by the thyroid gland, the effective half-life was determined to be approximately 6 days. The physical half-life of ^{131}I is 8.1 days. Calculate the biologic half-life.

$$\text{From } T_b = \frac{T_p \times T_e}{T_p - T_e} = \frac{8.1 \times 6}{8.1 - 6} = \frac{48.6}{2.1} = 23.1 \text{ days}$$

The biologic half-life of ^{24}Na in NaCl administered to an animal was found to be 12 hours. The physical half-life of ^{24}Na is 15 hours; calculate the effective half-life of ^{24}Na in this experiment.

$$\text{From } T_e = \frac{T_p \times T_b}{T_p + T_b} = \frac{15 \times 12}{15 + 12} = 6.7 \text{ hours.}$$

EXERCISES

A. The physical half-life of ^{59}Fe is 45 days. The biologic half-life of ^{59}Fe in the hemoglobin of an animal's erythrocytes was determined to be 62 days. What is the effective half-live of ^{59}Fe in this experiment?

B. The effective half-life of ^{32}P in a brain scan experiment in an animal was found to be approximately 10 days. The physical half-life of ^{32}P is 14.3 days. Calculate the biologic half-life of ^{32}P in this experiment.

9.4 SPECIFIC ACTIVITY

The classical definition of **specific activity** is the ratio of activity to the specific weight of a radionuclide. In most cases in nuclear medicine, however, the term refers to the number of millicuries per milliliter, mCi/ml, of solution. It may also be applied to compounds containing radioisotopes that are administered in scanning or therapy. The specific activity under these conditions is expressed in terms of the amount of activity per unit weight of the labelled compound as, for example, mCi per mg of Na ^{131}I. Calculations involving specific activity in solution are similar to those used in radioactive decay problems (Section 9.1). An equation that may be applied to calculate the specific weight of a sample of radioactive atoms is as follows:

$$W = 3.18 \times 10^{-13} \times A \times \text{At. wt.} \times t_{1/2}$$

where W is the weight in grams; A is the activity in mCi; At. wt. is the atomic weight of the atoms; and $t_{1/2}$ is the half-life in **hours.**

Examples

Calculate the weight of ^{131} I that contains 1.00 mCi of activity, and then calculate the specific activity of the sample. The half-life of ^{131} I is 8.1 days.

From $W = 3.18 \times 10^{-13} \times 1.00 \times 131 \times 8.1 \times 24\, h = 8.098 \times 10^{-9}$ g.

$$\text{Specific activity} = \frac{1.00\ \text{mCi}}{8.098 \times 10^{-9}\ \text{g}} = 1.23 \times 10^8\ \text{mCi/g or } 1.23 \times 10^5\ \text{Ci/g.}$$

A shipment of radioactive mercury, ^{197} Hg, had a specific activity of 300 μCi/mg on arrival Tuesday at 9 A.M. The half-life of ^{197}Hg is approximately 65 hours. At what time of the day and day of the week will the specific activity have dropped to 100 μCi/mg?

$$\text{From } \log \frac{I_o}{I} = 0.4343 \times \frac{0.693}{t_{1/2}} \times t, \quad \log \frac{300}{100} = 0.4343 \times \frac{0.693}{65} \times t,$$

or $\log 300 - \log 100 = 0.00463\ t$, and $2.4771 - 2.000 = 0.00463\ t$;

$$\text{therefore } t = \frac{0.4771}{0.00463} = 103 \text{ hours.}$$

Tuesday at 9 A.M. + 103 hours = Saturday at 4 P.M.

A solution of radioactive ^{32} P had a specific activity of 12 mCi/ml on August 4th. The half-life of ^{32} P is 14.3 days. Calculate the specific activity of the solution one month (30 days) later.

$$\text{From } \log \frac{I_o}{I} = 0.4343 \times \frac{0.693}{t_{1/2}} \times t = 0.4343 \times \frac{0.693}{14.3} \times 30 = 0.6314,$$

and $\log \frac{12}{I} = 0.6314$ or $\log 12 - \log I = 0.6314$;

therefore $\log I = \log 12 - 0.6314 = 1.0792 - 0.6314 = 0.4478$,

or $I = 2.8$ mCi/ml one month later.

EXERCISES

A. Calculate the weight of ^{59}Fe that contains 1.00 mCi of activity; then calculate the specific activity of the sample. The half-life of ^{59}Fe is 45 days. (Remember that half-life must be expressed in hours.)

B. A solution of radioactive ^{131}I has a specific activity of 250 μCi/ml on September 15th. The half-life of ^{131}I is 8.1 days. Calculate the specific activity of the solution on September 30th, 15 days later.

C. A shipment of radioactive strontium, ^{87m}Sr, had a specific activity of 75 mCi/mg on arrival Monday at 10 A.M. The half-life of ^{87m}Sr is 2.83 hours. At what time during the week would the specific activity be 10 mCi/mg?

9.5 SOLUTIONS OF RADIOISOTOPES

Radioisotopes are often supplied as labelled compounds dissolved in a solution. It is often desirable to know the relation between the activity, the concentration, and the volume of a solution. The concentration of a radioactive solution is usually expressed as mCi/ml or μCi/ml. When the activity and volume are known, the concentration is:

$$C = \frac{A}{V}$$

where A is expressed in mCi or μCi, and V is given in ml.

Examples

A vial contains 330 μCi of ^{131}I in 30 ml. What is the concentration?

From $C = \frac{A}{V}$, $C = \frac{330 \ \mu Ci}{30 \ ml} = 11 \ \mu Ci/ml$.

A vial contains 24 mCi of ^{57}Co in 30 ml. What is the concentration expressed in μCi/ml?

From $C = \frac{A}{V}$, $C = \frac{24 \ mCi}{30 \ ml} = 0.8 \ mCi/ml \times 1000 = 800 \ \mu Ci/ml$.

EXERCISES

A. A sample containing 75 μCi of ^{125}I is dissolved in water and made up to a volume of 5 ml. What is the concentration?

B. If a vial contains 2.0 mCi of ^{131}I in 12.5 ml of fluid, express the concentration in μCi/ml.

Often a vial of radioactive solution of known activity and volume, or concentration, is available. To administer the proper dose of radioactivity it is necessary to be able to calculate the volume that contains that amount of activity. The volume in milliliters is related to the desired activity and original concentration as follows:

$$V = \frac{A}{C}$$

where A is expressed in mCi or μCi, and C is given in mCi/ml or μCi/ml.

Examples

The concentration of ^{59}Fe in a vial is 65 mCi/ml. If a dose of 25 mCi is required, what volume of solution should be used?

$$\text{From } V = \frac{A}{C}, \quad V = \frac{25 \text{ mCi}}{65 \text{ mCi/ml}} = \frac{25 \text{ ml}}{65} = 0.385 \text{ ml.}$$

A vial contains 250 Ci of ^{57}Co in 2 ml of fluid. What volume should be withdrawn to obtain a dose of 150 μCi?

First calculate the original concentration from $C = \frac{A}{V}$:

$$C = \frac{250}{2} = 125 \ \mu\text{Ci/ml};$$

$$\text{then from } V = \frac{A}{C}, \quad V = \frac{150 \ \mu\text{Ci}}{125 \ \mu\text{Ci/ml}} = \frac{150 \text{ ml}}{125} = 1.2 \text{ ml.}$$

EXERCISES

C. A vial contains 12.5 mCi of ^{99} Tc in 5 ml of solution. What volume would be required for a dose of 3.5 mCi?

D. The concentration of ^{125} I in a vial is 150 μCi/ml. If a dose of 25 μCi is required, what volume of solution should be used?

E. A solution of 100 mCi of ^{131} I in 10 ml is diluted to a volume of 50 ml. What volume of the diluted solution is required for a dose of 15 mCi?

Helpful Hints. There are other ways to determine the half-life of a radioisotope in addition to calculation. There are several tables in textbooks and handbooks that list the half-life and decay constant of radioisotopes. If data similar to that shown in Table 10.3, p. 108, are available, the decay curve may be plotted on semilog paper (Figure 10.10), and the half-life determined graphically. The same decay curve could be used to determine the radioactivity remaining after any length of time. A similar graphical solution could be applied to the determination of the thickness of the half-value layer and the intensity of radiation that penetrates a sheet of absorbing material of varying thickness, if data for the preparation of the graph are available.

Another simple way to determine the activity of a specific radioisotope after a definite time period is by the use of **decay tables** found in radiation handbooks. An example of such tables is the ^{125}I decay table, found in the Appendix.

Radioactive decay factors may also be determined by use of the log-log scales on a slide rule. For example, to determine the decay factor for a definite time period, first set the hairline on 0.50 on the LL scale that contains the range which includes 0.50 (usually LL_2 or LL_0), and then slide the $T_{1/2}$ on the C scale under the hairline. (Example: 8.1 on the C scale for half-life of ^{131} I.) Move the hairline over the desired decay time on the C scale and read the fraction remaining on the appropriate LL scale (Example: After 4 days, the fraction reads 0.844, or 84.4 per cent.) Another example would be a solution of ^{99} Tc which had an activity of 50 mCi/ml at 9:30 A.M. If $T_{1/2}$ were 6 hours, what would be the specific activity at 11:30 A.M.? First set the hairline on 0.50 on the proper LL scale, and then slide 6 on the C scale under the hairline. Move the hairline over the 2 for 2 h, and read 0.926 or 92.6 per cent on the LL scale. Then 50 X 0.926 = 46.3 mCi/ml, the specific activity at 11:30 A.M. When using a slide rule in this fashion, if the desired decay time is off scale, move the hairline to the right or left C index that is on the slide rule scales, and then move the opposite C index to the hairline. Finally, move the hairline to the proper time and read the fraction off the proper LL scale.

10
The Preparation
of Graphs

THE *PRACTICAL OBJECTIVES* OF THIS CHAPTER ARE TO OBTAIN
AN UNDERSTANDING OF:

1. The equation of the graph for a straight line.

2. The proper construction of graphs for standards or calibration curves.

3. The use of graphs of radioactive decay curves.

4. The use of logarithmic and other scales to convert curves to straight-line relationships.

In high school and college mathematics courses the subject of functional relationships and graphs of functions is almost always covered. You may recall the simplest type of functional relationship in which y is directly proportional to x. This may be expressed as a general equation:

$$\frac{y}{x} = a \quad \text{or} \quad y = ax$$

This is the equation for a straight line since when x equals O, y is also equal to O. The greater the ratio of y/x, the steeper the line will be, and since $a = \frac{y}{x}$ a must represent the slope of the straight line.

The equation that is more relevant to the preparation of graphs in the laboratory is the linear function

$$y = ax + b$$

where a is the slope of the line and b is the intercept on the y axis. In the preparation of graphs we very often choose an intercept of 0, or b = 0, and the resultant straight line represents a linear function of y with respect to ax, as shown in the first equation. Since methods in the laboratory are calibrated by the preparation of a standard curve, x may represent the concentration of the standard solutions and y the absorbance readings obtained when the standards are run through the method. To illustrate the plotting of a graph through a series of points that correspond to successive values of x and y we may assume that the following values of x represent blood glucose values in mg/100 ml and y the absorbance of the respective solutions.

X	0	50	100	150	200	250
Y	0	0.151	0.303	0.449	0.602	0.748

It is common practice in the laboratory to plot concentration or time along the x or horizontal axis (abscissa) and change in absorbance, O.D., %T or changes in concentration with time on the y or vertical axis (ordinate).

10.1 THE CHOICE OF UNITS FOR THE COORDINATES

For practical purposes such as reading blood level values from a calibration curve it is essential to use most of the area on the graph paper in plotting the graph. This requires inspection of the graph paper to determine the number of major squares along both the ordinate and abscissa. For example, the commonly used millimeter square graph paper (Dietzen No. 341-M) has 18 major squares along the ordinate and 25 major squares along the abscissa. Along the x axis we would then choose each 5 major squares to represent 50 mg/dl blood glucose. Each major square on the y axis could represent an absorbance of 0.050, covering 15 major squares compared to the 25 major squares utilized on the x axis. When the graph is constructed in this fashion and the points for each set of x, y values are plotted, a straight line covering most of the area of the graph paper results (Figure 10.1). The wrong choice of units on either the ordinate or abscissa, as illustrated in Figure 10.2, could result in a graph of the function that would not only be awkward to read but would also produce inaccurate values.

Another example may be the preparation of a calibration curve for serum inorganic phosphorus. Values in the following tabulation were obtained for absorbance versus calibration standards concentration in mg/dl.

Conc. mg/dl (X)	0	2.0	4.0	6.0	8.0
Absorbance (Y)	0	0.198	0.401	0.603	0.799

If millimeter square graph paper (No. 341-M) is used, each five major squares on the abscissa could represent 2.0 mg/dl P and each major square on the ordinate 0.050 absorbance. The straight line obtained by joining the plotted points would then cover 20 squares on the abscissa and 16 squares on the ordinate, as shown in Figure 10.3.

Figure 10.1

Figure 10.2

Figure 10.3

In the preparation of graphs or calibration curves or in the graph of experimental data, the line does not always intercept the y axis at 0 or the origin. This may be caused by improper preparation or dilution of standard solutions, or may result from the presence of a contaminant that increases or decreases the absorbance of the experimental solutions. If we assume that Figure 10.1 represents a calibration curve for the glucose method in the laboratory as determined on a specific date, and the following data were obtained in the preparation of another calibration curve for this method one week later, the two calibrations would appear as shown in Figure 10.4.

Table 10.1

Conc., mg/dl	50	100	150	200	250
Absorbance	0.201	0.353	0.499	0.652	0.798

The two curves obviously represent a linear relationship between the absorbance and concentration of glucose, yet the 5-12-75 curve is parallel to that of 5-5-75 and does not pass through the origin. This situation suggests that a common dilution error has been made in the preparation of the standard solutions that correspond to the five concentrations in Table 10.1.

Figure 10.4

10.2. THE PREPARATION OF STANDARD CURVES

Although we have already discussed standard curves and used values from standard solutions of glucose and phosphorus to illustrate the graphs of linear functions, the subject is worth exploring in greater detail. When setting up a new or modified spectrophotometric method in the laboratory, the first step should involve **the construction of a calibration curve**. The curve should cover the entire range of concentrations met in practice, and it is essential to duplicate experimental conditions that will be employed in the routine analysis of specimens. Assuming that accurate standards are prepared and that the procedure is carried out with satisfactory technique, the spectrophotometric readings shown in Table 10.2 may result.

TABLE 10.2

Standard concentration (mg/dl)	%T	Absorbance
0	100.0	0.000
10	80.3	0.095
25	57.7	0.239
50	33.2	0.480
75	19.2	0.718
100	11.1	0.960

The two types of readings given in the above tabulation are obtained from instruments and scales commonly encountered in clinical laboratories. They are related to each other as follows:

$$\text{Absorbance} = 2 - \log \% \, T$$

At least three types of standard curves can be prepared from the above data plotting concentration on the abscissa versus spectrophotometric readings on the ordinate. Figure 10.5 illustrates a plot of % T (% transmission) versus concentration. This type of plot is not recommended for routine use for several reasons. The relationship is not linear, nor is it apparent from the curve whether the readings obtained from the method follows Beer's law (see Chapter 8, p. 81). Several concentration points must be obtained to construct a smooth curve, and errors of measurement are more difficult to assess. When % T values are plotted on one cycle semilog paper, a linear relationship between the readings and the concentration is evident, as seen in Figure 10.6. The direct and linear relationship between absorbance. and the concentration is shown in Figure 10.7. **This type of plot is recommended for routine use in the laboratory.** It produces a straight line with a positive slope in which an increase in concentration results in an increase of absorbance. The relationship is linear and a positive test of Beer's law is obtained from the readings. Once the standard curve is prepared for a method, it may be routinely checked by the use of a reagent blank plus two standard solutions, which represent the concentration of the highest standard and one-half the concentration of that standard in the accurate range of the method. In the standard curve shown in Figure 10.7, for example, the zero concentration or reagent blank, the 50 mg/dl and the 100 mg/dl standards would be used to check the calibration curve of the method.

Figure 10.5

Figure 10.6

Figure 10.7

The current trend by laboratory instrument manufactures is to produce **spectrophotometers with linear absorbance scales, digital displays or print-out systems.** These instruments will obviate the conversion of % T to absorbance values and simplify the preparation of linear calibration curves. For laboratories that use instruments containing only a % T scale the Table in the Appendix permits ready conversion of such readings to absorbance values.

10.3 GRAPHS OF RADIOLOGIC FUNCTIONS

In the last section we have observed the use of one-cycle semilog paper to obtain a **linear relationship** between % T values and concentration. Another common example of the use of **logarithmic relationships** may be found in the preparation of graphs to illustrate the course of radioactive decay of an element. Radioactive iodine, ^{131}I, has a half-life of approximately 8 days. Values for the approximate strength or radioactive decay of ^{131}I are shown in Table 10.3

Table 10.3

Time (days)	Approx. strength of ^{131}I (per cent)	Logarithm of approx. strength of ^{131}I
0	100	2.0
8	50	1.7
16	25	1.4
24	12.5	1.1
32	6.25	0.8
40	3.13	0.5

The values in the second column are obviously obtained by dividing each successive value by two, whereas the third column represents approximate logarithm values obtained by subtracting (division) the log of 2 (approximately 0.3) from each successive value.

If the values for the strength of ^{131}I in the second column are plotted against time in days, the curve in Figure 10.8 is obtained.

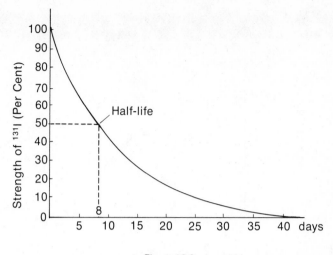

Figure 10.8

This curve is not suitable for quantitative assessment of radioactive decay even if it was prepared from accurate values for the strength of ^{131} I. There are two solutions to the problem. One is to plot the logarithms of the strength of ^{131} I with time as shown in Figure 10.9, and the other, more convenient, method is to plot the strength of ^{131}I on the logarithm scale of two-cycle semilog paper, as shown in Figure 10.10. It should be apparent that the origin on the ordinate of semilog paper starts with 1.0 or 10 (see Figure 10.10) or possibly 0.1, and that only the first four values in the second column may be plotted on a one-cycle semilog paper.

Figure 10.9

Figure 10.10

Expressions other than logarithms may be used to convert relationships from a curved-line form to a straight-line form in the preparation of graphs. The biochemist uses a reciprocal relationship in plotting the velocity of an enzyme reaction against the concentration of the substrate to obtain a linear relation. This is the Lineweaver-Burk plot of $\frac{1}{v}$ versus $\frac{1}{[S]}$. In measuring the dose rate at various distances from an x-ray source, Table 10.4, the radiologist is confronted

Table 10.4

Distance from x-ray source (feet)	$\dfrac{1}{\text{Distance}^2}$	Dose rate (R/min)
2	0.2500	90
3	0.1111	40
4	0.0625	22.5
5	0.0400	14.5
6	0.0277	10
7	0.0204	7.5
8	0.0156	6

with an awkward curve when the dose rates in R/min are plotted against distance in feet, as shown in Figure 10.11. When the dose rate is plotted against the reciprocal of the distance squared, Figure 10.12, a linear relationship is obtained. The mathematician would say that the dose rate is inversely proportional to the distance squared.

Figure 10.11

Figure 10.12

10.4. THE GLUCOSE TOLERANCE CURVE

Glucose tolerance tests are often run in a clinical laboratory. A blood specimen is drawn from a fasted patient and 75 to 100 grams of glucose is given by mouth, followed by the drawing of additional blood specimens at specific time intervals. A graph illustrating the glucose tolerance curve of the patient would be constructed by plotting changes in blood glucose with time. The results of such a tolerance test are shown in the following tabulation.

Time (hours) (X)	0	0.5	1.0	1.5	2.0	2.5
Blood Glucose (mg/dl) (Y)	70	90	120	150	130	100

On millimeter square graph paper (No. 341-M) each five major squares on the abscissa could represent 0.5 hour and each five major squares on the ordinate 50 mg/dl blood glucose. The resultant curve would obviously not be a straight line and would not start at zero on the ordinate (Figure 10.13). It would follow the patient's blood sugar level starting at 70, rising to 150 at 1.5 hours, then dropping to 100 mg/dl at 2.5 hours after the ingestion of the glucose.

EXERCISES

1. Explain the terms in the following equation: $y = ax + b$

2. Which two terms in the above equation are most important in the clinical laboratory? Explain.

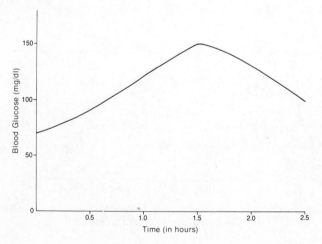

Figure 10.13

3. In the preparation of a calibration curve in the laboratory the following data was collected.

Conc., mg/dl	0	2.5	5.0	7.5	10.0
Absorbance	0	0.198	0.401	0.595	0.798

Plot the points and construct the standard curve from these values.

4. Data for the preparation of a calibration curve for serum inorganic phosphorus was as follows:

Conc., mg/dl	2.0	4.0	6.0	8.0
Absorbance	0.301	0.498	0.702	0.901

Plot the calibration curve from the above data. Is this a satisfactory standard curve? Explain.

5. The only spectrophotometer in the laboratory had a scale graduated in % T. The readings obtained for a series of standard solutions were as follows:

Conc., mg/dl	0	5	10	25	50
%T	100.0	81.5	66.5	37.5	14.0

Plot the standard curve as absorbance versus concentration values.

6. The half-life of radon is approximately 4 days. Construct a graph that illustrates a linear relationship between the strength of the radon after 4, 8, 12, 16, and 20 days.

11
Quality Control Statistics

THE *PRACTICAL OBJECTIVES* OF THIS CHAPTER ARE TO OBTAIN
AN UNDERSTANDING OF:

1. The value of the mean, the standard deviation, and coefficient of variation in quality control statistics.

2. The use and construction of quality control charts.

3. The value of the chi-square test in instrument control.

4. The use of graphs in method comparison studies.

5. The types of laboratory errors and their recognition.

6. The value of the t test in the comparison of methods and experimental regimes.

Quality control methods are commonly employed in the modern clinical laboratory to ensure the constant production of reliable results. There are many expressions, borrowed from statistics, that are used to maintain confidence in analytic values. A comparison, for example, of the meaning of the terms accuracy, precision and reliability may help set the stage for a discussion of the application of statistics to laboratory mathematics.

The **accuracy** of a method for the determination of a substance refers to the agreement of the results with the true value for that substance in the specimen. In the clinical laboratory it is not always possible to obtain primary standards that represent the true value of a constituent, and reference standards are often used. The **precision** of a method refers to its ability to produce a series of results that agree very closely with each other. If ten determinations of a single constituent result in values that are in close agreement, the method has a high degree of precision. This obviously does not mean that the method is necessarily accurate since there are many examples of methods for glucose, urea and calcium that exhibit precision and yet do not measure the true value for the particular constituent. The **reliability** of a method is a measure of its ability to achieve both accuracy and precision. A reliable method would therefore be one that consistently produced accurate and precise results in the determination of a laboratory constituent.

11.1 MEAN, STANDARD DEVIATION, AND COEFFICIENT OF VARIATION

Blood glucose values obtained by the use of tungstic acid protein-free filtrates (Folin-Wu) and by a glucose oxidase "true glucose" method may be used to illustrate statistical calculations. Ten determinations were run by each method on the same specimen and the values are shown in Table 11.1 The **mean value** for each method, X, equals the sum of the ten values divided by N, the number of individual results or:

$$\text{Mean} = \overline{X} = \frac{\Sigma x}{N}$$

The **range of values** is an expression of the precision or repeatability of the method. A very commonly used measure of precision is called the standard deviation, s, which represents the scattering of values around the mean and is related to distribution curves and quality control charts. The **standard deviation** equals the square root of the sum of the squared differences from the mean divided by one less than the number of determinations.

$$s = \sqrt{\frac{\Sigma (X - \overline{X})^2}{N - 1}}$$

Another method that is used to compare the results of two sets of data is the calculation of the **coefficient of variation**. This term expresses the scattering of results as percentages of the mean and may be used to compare values of different magnitudes and different units. The coefficient of variation, C. V., may be expressed as follows:

$$\text{C. V.} = \frac{s}{\overline{X}} \times 100$$

Calculations for these expressions are illustrated for the two sets of blood glucose values in Table 11.1.

From the calculated results for the two methods we would conclude that the Folin-Wu type method demonstrated the most precision, i.e., lower standard deviation and coefficient of variation, whereas the true glucose method was more accurate since the values grouped around the true glucose value.

EXERCISES

A. A serum specimen was analyzed ten times for its chloride content. The following values, expressed in milliequivalents/liter, were obtained: 106, 103, 105, 102, 105, 104, 106, 103, 102, 104. Calculate the standard deviation.

TABLE 11.1

Folin-Wu glucose mg/dl	Deviation from mean	Deviation squared	True glucose mg/dl	Deviation from mean	Deviation squared
98	−1	1	87	+1	1
101	+2	4	85	−1	1
99	0	0	86	0	0
97	−2	4	83	−3	9
98	−1	1	89	+3	9
102	+3	9	84	−2	4
99	0	0	86	0	0
101	+2	4	87	+1	1
98	−1	1	85	−1	1
97	−2	4	88	+2	4
990		28	860		30

Mean $= \overline{X} = \dfrac{\Sigma X}{N} = \dfrac{990}{10} = 99$ mg/dl $\qquad$ Mean $= \overline{X} = \dfrac{\Sigma X}{N} = \dfrac{860}{10} = 86$ mg/dl

Range 97 – 102 mg/dl $\qquad\qquad$ Range 83 – 89 mg/dl

$$\text{Standard deviation } s = \sqrt{\frac{\Sigma (X - \overline{X})^2}{N-1}}$$

$s = \sqrt{\dfrac{28}{9}} = \sqrt{3.11} = 1.76$ mg/dl $\qquad\qquad s = \sqrt{\dfrac{30}{9}} = \sqrt{3.33} = 1.83$ mg/dl

$$\text{C. V.} = \frac{s}{\overline{X}} \times 100$$

C. V. $= \dfrac{1.76}{99} \times 100 = 1.78$ per cent $\qquad$ C. V. $= \dfrac{1.83}{86} \times 100 = 2.13$ per cent

B. A serum specimen was obtained from a male laboratory technician and a female laboratory technician. Each specimen was analyzed ten times for uric acid content with the following results: Male 6.2, 6.0, 6.0, 6.4, 5.9, 6.1, 6.4, 5.8, 6.3, 5.9. Female 5.5, 5.7, 5.9, 5.7, 5.6, 5.8, 5.6, 5.6, 5.9, 5.7. Calculate the standard deviation and coefficient of variation for each set of values.

Helpful Hints. The standard deviation for a set of values may be calculated in another fashion which may represent a simplification of the method used in Table 11.1. The equation is as follows:

$$s = \sqrt{\frac{\Sigma (x^2) - (\Sigma x)^2}{N - 1}}$$

As an example, apply this equation to the calculation of s for the true glucose values in Table 11.1. Using a slide rule or electronic calculator, the x^2 values are as follows: 7569, 7225, 7396, 6889, 7921, 7056, 7396, 7569, 7225, and 7744. The $\Sigma (x^2) = 73990$; the $\frac{(\Sigma x)^2}{N} = \frac{(860)^2}{10} = 73960$; then

$$s = \sqrt{\frac{73990 - 73960}{9}} = \sqrt{\frac{30}{9}} = 1.83 \text{ mg/dl,}$$

which is the same value as that shown in Table 11.1. Applying this method to the Folin-Wu glucose values results in an s of 1.76, which again is the same value as calculated in Table 11.1.

11.2 QUALITY CONTROL CHARTS

In quality control systems the deviation of a value from the true value and the distribution of the values around the mean are important considerations. If a single constituent is determined in the serum of a large group of individuals and the **frequency of occurrence** of each value is plotted, the result is a normal or gaussian distribution curve (Figure 11.1).

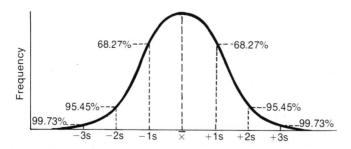

Figure 11.1

The mean value corresponds to the peak in the distribution of results in a **normal distribution curve**. If the standard deviation is calculated for a large series of results the percentage would be as follows:

$$\pm 1.0 \text{ standard deviation from the mean } 68.27\%$$
$$\pm 2.0 \text{ standard deviation from the mean } 95.45\%$$
$$\pm 3.0 \text{ standard deviation from the mean } 99.73\%$$

A **quality control chart** usually represents the distribution of values of a reference standard as follows:

```
+3s  _ _ _ _ _ _ _ _ _ _ _ _ _ _ _ _ _ _ _ _ _ _ _ _ _ _ _ _ _ _
+2s  _ _ _ _ _ _ _ _ _ _ _ _ _ _ _ _ _ _ _ _ _ _ _ _ _ _ _ _ _ _
+1s  _ _ _ _ _ _ _ _ _ _ _ _ _ _ _ _ _ _ _ _ _ _ _ _ _ _ _ _ _ _
 X̄   _____
-1s  _ _ _ _ _ _ _ _ _ _ _ _ _ _ _ _ _ _ _ _ _ _ _ _ _ _ _ _ _ _
-2s  _ _ _ _ _ _ _ _ _ _ _ _ _ _ _ _ _ _ _ _ _ _ _ _ _ _ _ _ _ _
-3s  _ _ _ _ _ _ _ _ _ _ _ _ _ _ _ _ _ _ _ _ _ _ _ _ _ _ _ _ _ _
```

As an example, we may represent the values that were calculated for the true glucose method on such a chart (Figure 11.2). The mean value was 86 mg/dl, and s was 1.8 mg/dl.

Glucose mg/dl

Figure 11.2

In most laboratories the acceptable limits of precision for a method used in quality control is ± 2.0 s, which includes 95.5 per cent of all the values obtained for the reference standard.

Quality control charts are often used to monitor the daily counting of a radioisotope check source. Replicate values and standard deviation data for a ^{125} I check source in a gamma counter are shown in Table 11.2

TABLE 11.2

Radioactive Counts	Deviation from Mean	Deviation Squared
164391	130	16900
164593	332	110224
164260	1	1
164076	185	34225
163732	529	279841
164042	219	47961
164468	207	42849
164470	209	43681
164183	78	6084
164390	129	16641
1642605		598407

$$\text{Mean} = \overline{x} = \frac{1642605}{10} = 164261 \text{ counts}$$

$$s = \sqrt{\frac{598407}{9}} = 258$$

$$1s = \pm258$$

$$2s = \pm516$$

$$3s = \pm774$$

A quality control chart based on the data in Table 11.2 with daily counts of the ^{125}I check source for 20 days is shown in Figure 11.3.

Figure 11.3

EXERCISE

A. Construct a quality control chart for the radioactive counts in Table 11.2, including ±2.0 standard deviations as the limit of control.

11.3 THE CHI-SQUARE TEST

A task-oriented application of statistics involves the use of the chi-square test to monitor the proper operation of radioisotope counting equipment. The test determines the conformance of the measured counts to an assumed Poisson distribution of radioactive counts. The chi-square valve, χ^2, may be calculated as follows:

$$\chi^2 = \frac{\Sigma (x_i - \bar{x})^2}{\bar{x}}$$

where x_i represents each of N individual measurements and x is the average value.

A test of the counting instrument is usually carried out after a background check and an E-dial calibration. Ten or twenty one-minute counts are read using a 20 kev window centered about the photopeak. The chi-square value is calculated from the readings and the probability value, p, is determined from the information in Table 11.3

Table 11.3

No. of Readings	Chi-Square Values						
	0.99*	0.95	0.90	0.50	0.10	0.05	0.01
10	2.088	3.325	4.168	8.343	14.684	16.919	21.666
20	7.633	10.117	11.651	18.338	27.204	30.144	36.191
	0.99*	0.95	0.90	0.50	0.10	0.05	0.01

*Corresponding p values.

If the p value is less than 0.10 or greater than 0.90, faulty instrument performance is indicated. A p value between 0.10 and 0.90, however, indicates that the instrument is operating properly and the observed distribution of counts corresponds to the assumed Poisson distribution. As an example, the data in Table 11.4 were obtained from ten one-minute counts in a gamma counter using a 15 to 100 kev window, a principal photopeak of 35 kev, and a ^{125}I check source.

TABLE 11.4

x_i	$(x_i - \bar{x})$	$(x_i - \bar{x})^2$
165183	922	850084
164160	101	10201
163862	399	159201
164121	140	19600
164390	129	16641
164183	78	6084
164470	209	43681
164468	207	42849
164042	219	47961
163732	529	279841
1642611		1476143

$$\bar{x} = \frac{1642611}{10} = 164261 \qquad \chi^2 = \frac{1476143}{164261} = 8.99$$

The value for χ^2 of 8.99 falls about halfway between a p value of 0.10 and 0.90; therefore, the instrument is operating properly.

EXERCISE

A. Using the same instrument and conditions as outlined for the example in Table 11.4, the following ten one-minute counts were obtained.

164568	164471	163936	164671	164397
164809	164270	164266	164686	164622

Calculate χ^2 and interpret the meaning of the p value.

11.4 METHOD COMPARISON STATISTICS

The introduction of new methods of analysis is frequently considered by the staff of a laboratory in order to improve or simplify existing analytical methodology. Before adoption of such a method it should be compared to an existing method or reference method in the laboratory. Such comparison studies yield paired values from the same serum specimen that may be used for statistical treatment of the data. A simple comparison of the results obtained by the two methods is to plot the values from one method on the ordinate and the values from the other on the abscissa. The units on the graph paper should be chosen to accommodate a 45°—angle line through the points on the curve. The total graph would therefore be close to a square shape, since the best linear fit of the data would follow a line from the lower left-hand corner to the upper right-hand corner of the graph.

As an example, let us assume that four new methods for serum glucose are being compared with an existing method in the laboratory. Paired samples from standard solutions of glucose of increasing concentrations were run by all methods; the values obtained are shown in Table 11.5.

TABLE 11.5

Specimen	Methods for Serum Glucose (mg/dl)				
	Existing	A	B	C	D
1	0	1	11	2	1
2	25	24	33	30	24
3	52	49	60	56	50
4	73	75	84	70	76
5	101	98	110	93	103
6	124	126	137	134	127
7	149	151	159	145	155
8	176	173	186	170	180
9	198	201	210	209	208
10	222	225	236	232	231
11	246	251	258	243	261
12	277	274	287	278	288
13	301	297	309	292	315
14	327	328	334	319	345
15	348	353	361	358	372

When the values from method A are plotted on the ordinate against the values from the existing method on the abscissa, the graph shown in Figure 11.4 is obtained.

Figure 11.4

It is readily apparent from the points on the graph, sometimes called a *scatter diagram* or *scattergram,* that a close linear correlation exists between the results obtained from method A and those from the existing method.

11.5 USE OF SCATTERGRAMS IN THE ASSESSMENT OF TYPES OF ERRORS

The points along the line in Figure 11.4 illustrate a type of error known as *no error,* or a very small methodologic error. When the values from method B in Table 11.5 are plotted against those from the existing method, as shown in Figure 11.5, a *constant error* is illustrated.

The points on this line indicate a constant added increment of serum glucose or contaminants being measured in method B. (See also Figure 10.4 as an additional example of this type of error.)

Plotting the values from method C against those from the existing method, as shown in Figure 11.6, points out a common error called a *random error.*

When values from method D are plotted against those from the existing method, a type of error known as a *proportional error* is illustrated, as shown in Figure 11.7

Figure 11.5

Figure 11.6

Figure 11.7

In this type of error the values either increase or decrease proportionately as the concentration of the specimen increases.

The points on Figures 11.5 through 11.7 are not extreme examples of the different types of errors, but should illustrate the concept of laboratory error. At times the points represent a more severe scattergram. In any case, using a clear plastic ruler to fit the best line to the curve is usually sufficient for practical purposes. If a laboratory computer is available, the values may be fed into a computer program that will draw the graph and calculate the best fitting line by the method of least squares. An equation for the line will result that assigns a value to the y intercept and to the slope of the line. Manual calculations by the least squares method are too complex to be presented in the present discussion.

11.6 The *t* TEST OF SIGNIFICANCE OF DIFFERENCE BETWEEN TWO MEANS

There are many occasions in the laboratory when it is important to know if there is a significant difference in the results obtained by two different methods for the same constituent. In such cases, the *t* test may be used. It applies when the results from a new method are compared to those obtained from the method in common use in the laboratory. The t test may also be used, for instance, to test data obtained from male subjects versus female subjects in the same study, or to test the significance of the difference between values obtained from a group of subjects during a control period compared to results obtained during an experimental period (e.g., change of diet, effect of treatment, or effect of drugs).

The statistic t is defined as the ratio of difference between two means to the standard deviation of this difference, or

$$t = \frac{\bar{d}}{S_d} \sqrt{n}$$

where $\bar{d}$ is the mean of the differences between the two methods or parameters of comparison, n is the number of pairs of values, and S_d is the standard deviation of the differences, or

$$S_d = \sqrt{\frac{\Sigma (d^2) - (\Sigma d)^2}{n - 1}}$$

A table of t values may be found in the Appendix. If the calculated value of t exceeds that shown in the t Table, the difference is significant at the probability chosen. The limits of significance commonly chosen are the 95 per cent limits.

As an example of the value of the t test, we will consider the data in Table 11.6, which represents total protein values in the serum of subjects during a drug-free control period compared to the values obtained after one day, two days, and three days of a drug regimen (ten 5-grain aspirin tablets a day).

Examples

To determine if the drug regimen affects the total protein values, we are looking for a significant difference between each day on drugs versus the control protein values. In comparing values for the first day against those of the control day, the calculations would be as follows:

From Table 11.6,

$$\Sigma d = -1.7; \; \Sigma d^2 = 2.07, \; n = 22; \; \bar{d} = \frac{-1.7}{22} = -0.077; \; (\Sigma d)^2 = (-1.7)^2 = 2.89$$

$$S_d = \sqrt{\frac{\Sigma d^2 - \frac{(\Sigma d)^2}{n}}{n - 1}} = \sqrt{\frac{2.07 - \frac{2.89}{22}}{21}} = \sqrt{\frac{2.07 - 0.13}{21}} = \sqrt{\frac{1.94}{21}} = 0.304$$

$$\text{and } t = \frac{\bar{d}}{S_d} \sqrt{n} = \frac{-0.077 \times 4.69}{0.304} = -1.19$$

From the t Table (Appendix), $t = 2.08$ for 21 degrees of freedom $(n - 1)$ at the 95 per cent level. Since the t value of -1.19 for the first day compared to the control values does not exceed 2.08, the difference between the total protein values for the two days is not significant.

A further example would be to calculate the t value for the second day against the control values.

From Table 11.6,

$$\Sigma d = -2.7; \; \Sigma d^2 = 1.65; n = 22; \bar{d} = \frac{-2.7}{22} = -0.123; (\Sigma d)^2 = 7.29$$

TABLE 11.6

Subject	Control Value	First Day d*	d²	Second Day Value	d*	d²	Third Day Value	d*	d²
1	7.9	+ 0.1	.01	7.5	− 0.4	.16	7.9	0	0
2	8.2	− 0.1	.01	7.8	− 0.4	.16	7.9	− 0.3	.09
3	7.1	+ 0.5	.25	7.4	+ 0.3	.09	7.2	+ 0.1	.01
4	7.7	7.7 0	0	7.7	0	0	7.5	− 0.2	.04
5	7.5	− 0.1	.01	7.4	− 0.1	.01	7.4	− 0.1	.01
6	7.5	− 0.5	.25	7.1	− 0.4	.16	7.4	− 0.1	.01
7	7.0	+ 0.1	.01	7.0	0	0	6.9	− 0.1	.01
8	8.1	− 0.1	.01	8.0	− 0.1	.01	7.8	− 0.3	.09
9	7.5	− 0.3	.09	7.4	− 0.1	.01	7.5	0	0
10	7.8	+ 0.3	.09	7.7	− 0.1	.01	7.4	− 0.4	.16
11	7.7	− 0.6	.36	6.9	− 0.8	.64	6.9	− 0.8	.64
12	7.8	+ 0.1	.01	7.9	+ 0.1	.01	7.7	− 0.1	.01
13	7.8	+ 0.1	.01	7.8	0	0	7.7	− 0.1	.01
14	7.6	− 0.3	.09	7.2	− 0.4	.16	7.2	− 0.4	.16
15	7.2	+ 0.3	.09	7.1	− 0.1	.01	7.1	− 0.1	.01
16	7.1	− 0.4	.16	7.1	0	0	6.4	− 0.7	.49
17	7.3	+ 0.3	.09	7.3	0	0	7.1	− 0.2	.04
18	8.4	− 0.6	.36	8.2	− 0.2	.04	8.0	− 0.4	.16
19	7.5	7.5 0	0	7.8	+ 0.3	.09	7.6	+ 0.1	.01
20	7.5	7.5 0	0	7.3	− 0.2	.04	7.5	0	0
21	7.5	− 0.4	.16	7.6	+ 0.1	.01	7.3	− 0.2	.04
22	7.9	− 0.1	.01	7.7	− 0.2	.04	7.8	− 0.1	.01
		− 1.7	2.07		− 2.7	1.65		− 4.4	2.00

$\Sigma d = -1.7$ $\quad$ $\Sigma d = -2.7$ $\quad$ $\Sigma d = -4.4$

$\Sigma d^2 = 2.07$ $\quad$ $\Sigma d^2 = 1.65$ $\quad$ $\Sigma d^2 = 2.00$

*The d values for each day represent the difference between the total protein values on the control day and the values on the first, second, or third day of the drug regimen.

$$S_d = \sqrt{\dfrac{\Sigma d^2 - (\Sigma d)^2}{n-1}} = \sqrt{\dfrac{1.65 - \dfrac{7.29}{22}}{21}} = \sqrt{\dfrac{1.65 - 0.33}{21}} = \sqrt{\dfrac{1.32}{21}} = 0.251$$

$$t = \dfrac{\bar{d}}{S_d}\sqrt{n} = \dfrac{-0.123 \times 4.69}{0.251} = -2.30$$

The total protein values on the second day are therefore significantly lower than those on the control day, since the t value of -2.30 exceeds 2.08 at the 95 per cent level.

EXERCISES

A. Calculate the t value for the total protein levels on the third day of the drug regimen compared to those of the control day.

B. In a comparison of paired samples by two methods for total protein in the serum, the following results were obtained:

Method A: 7.2, 7.0, 7.3, 7.1, 7.7, 6.9, 8.2, 7.7, 7.7, 7.6, 7.0, 8.0, 7.2, 7.8, 7.7, 7.3, 6.8, 7.2, 7.0, 7.3

Method B: 7.2, 7.2, 7.0, 7.1, 7.3, 6.7, 7.3, 7.7, 7.3, 7.2, 6.8, 7.3, 6.7, 7.0, 7.6, 7.0, 6.8, 7.3, 7.0, 7.8

Calculate the t value for method B against method A. Is the t value significant at the 95 per cent level? Hint: Arrange the values in tabular form similar to Table 11.6 to determine d and d^2 and Σd and Σd^2. From the t Table in the Appendix, $t = 2.093$ for 19 degrees of freedom at the 95 per cent level.

ADDITIONAL EXERCISES

1. Construct a quality control chart for the uric acid values for the male laboratory technician (Exercise B, p. 73) including ± 2.0 standard deviations as the limit of control.

2. A pooled serum sample was analyzed 20 times for its urea nitrogen content. Values in mg/dl were obtained as follows: 12.2, 12.4, 12.0, 12.5, 12.3, 12.3, 12.6, 12.0, 12.5, 12.2, 12.4, 12.1, 12.6, 12.2, 12.3, 12.2, 12.5, 12.4, 12.4, 12.6. Construct a quality control chart from these values including ± 2.0 standard deviations from the mean.

3. Construct a quality control chart for the Folin-Wu glucose values in Table 11.1. Plot the ten values and indicate those which fall outside the ± 2.0 s limits.

4. In a further experiment, using the same instrument and conditions as outlined for the example in Table 11.3, the following 10 1-minute counts were obtained for another specimen:

45515	45599	45574	45079	45392
45370	45341	45718	45510	45152

Calculate χ^2 and interpret the meaning of the p value.

Appendix

FOUR PLACE LOGARITHMS *

											Average differences								
x	0	1	2	3	4	5	6	7	8	9	1	2	3	4	5	6	7	8	9
10	0000	0043	0086	0128	0170	0212	0253	0294	0334	0374	4	8	12	17	21	25	29	33	37
11	0414	0453	0492	0531	0569	0607	0645	0682	0719	0755	4	8	11	15	19	23	26	30	34
12	0792	0828	0864	0899	0934	0969	1004	1038	1072	1106	3	7	10	14	17	21	24	28	31
13	1139	1173	1206	1239	1271	1303	1335	1367	1399	1430	3	6	10	13	16	19	23	26	29
14	1461	1492	1523	1553	1584	1614	1644	1673	1703	1732	3	6	9	12	15	18	21	24	27
15	1761	1790	1818	1847	1875	1903	1931	1959	1987	2014	3	6	8	11	14	17	20	22	25
16	2041	2068	2095	2122	2148	2175	2201	2227	2253	2279	3	5	8	11	13	16	18	21	24
17	2304	2330	2355	2380	2405	2430	2455	2480	2504	2529	2	5	7	10	12	15	17	20	22
18	2553	2577	2601	2625	2648	2672	2695	2718	2742	2765	2	5	7	9	12	14	16	19	21
19	2788	2810	2833	2856	2878	2900	2923	2945	2967	2989	2	4	7	9	11	13	16	18	20
20	3010	3032	3054	3075	3096	3118	3139	3160	3181	3201	2	4	6	8	11	13	15	17	19
21	3222	3243	3263	3284	3304	3324	3345	3365	3385	3404	2	4	6	8	10	12	14	16	18
22	3424	3444	3464	3483	3502	3522	3541	3560	3579	3598	2	4	6	8	10	12	14	15	17
23	3617	3636	3655	3674	3692	3711	3729	3747	3766	3784	2	4	6	7	9	11	13	15	17
24	3802	3820	3838	3856	3874	3892	3909	3927	3945	3962	2	4	5	7	9	11	12	14	16
25	3979	3997	4014	4031	4048	4065	4082	4099	4116	4133	2	3	5	7	9	10	12	14	15
26	4150	4166	4183	4200	4216	4232	4249	4265	4281	4298	2	3	5	7	8	10	11	13	15
27	4314	4330	4346	4362	4378	4393	4409	4425	4440	4456	2	3	5	6	8	9	11	13	14
28	4472	4487	4502	4518	4533	4548	4564	4579	4594	4609	2	3	5	6	8	9	11	12	14
29	4624	4639	4654	4669	4683	4698	4713	4728	4742	4757	1	3	4	6	7	9	10	12	13
30	4771	4786	4800	4814	4829	4843	4857	4871	4886	4900	1	3	4	6	7	9	10	11	13
31	4914	4928	4942	4955	4969	4983	4997	5011	5024	5038	1	3	4	6	7	8	10	11	12
32	5051	5065	5079	5092	5105	5119	5132	5145	5159	5172	1	3	4	5	7	8	9	11	12
33	5185	5198	5211	5224	5237	5250	5263	5276	5289	5302	1	3	4	5	6	8	9	10	12
34	5315	5328	5340	5353	5366	5378	5391	5403	5416	5428	1	3	4	5	6	8	9	10	11
35	5441	5453	5465	5478	5490	5502	5514	5527	5539	5551	1	2	4	5	6	7	9	10	11
36	5563	5575	5587	5599	5611	5623	5635	5647	5658	5670	1	2	4	5	6	7	8	10	11
37	5682	5694	5705	5717	5729	5740	5752	5763	5775	5786	1	2	3	5	6	7	8	9	10
38	5798	5809	5821	5832	5843	5855	5866	5877	5888	5899	1	2	3	5	6	7	8	9	10
39	5911	5922	5933	5944	5955	5966	5977	5988	5999	6010	1	2	3	4	5	7	8	9	10
40	6021	6031	6042	6053	6064	6075	6085	6096	6107	6117	1	2	3	4	5	6	8	9	10
41	6128	6138	6149	6160	6170	6180	6191	6201	6212	6222	1	2	3	4	5	6	7	8	9
42	6232	6243	6253	6263	6274	6284	6294	6304	6314	6325	1	2	3	4	5	6	7	8	9
43	6335	6345	6355	6365	6375	6385	6395	6405	6415	6425	1	2	3	4	5	6	7	8	9
44	6435	6444	6454	6464	6474	6484	6493	6503	6513	6522	1	2	3	4	5	6	7	8	9
45	6532	6542	6551	6561	6571	6580	6590	6599	6609	6618	1	2	3	4	5	6	7	8	9
46	6628	6637	6646	6656	6665	6675	6684	6693	6702	6712	1	2	3	4	5	6	7	7	8
47	6721	6730	6739	6749	6758	6767	6776	6785	6794	6803	1	2	3	4	5	5	6	7	8
48	6812	6821	6830	6839	6848	6857	6866	6875	6884	6893	1	2	3	4	5	5	6	7	8
49	6902	6911	6920	6928	6937	6946	6955	6964	6972	6981	1	2	3	4	4	5	6	7	8
50	6990	6998	7007	7016	7024	7033	7042	7050	7059	7067	1	2	3	3	4	5	6	7	8
51	7076	7084	7093	7101	7110	7118	7126	7135	7143	7152	1	2	3	3	4	5	6	7	8
52	7160	7168	7177	7185	7193	7202	7210	7218	7226	7235	1	2	2	3	4	5	6	7	7
53	7243	7251	7259	7267	7275	7284	7292	7300	7308	7316	1	2	2	3	4	5	6	6	7
54	7324	7332	7340	7348	7356	7364	7372	7380	7388	7396	1	2	2	3	4	5	6	6	7
x	0	1	2	3	4	5	6	7	8	9	1	2	3	4	5	6	7	8	9

*From Stevenson, R.: Saunders Short Tables, Philadelphia, W. B. Saunders Company, 1967.

FOUR PLACE LOGARITHMS*

x	0	1	2	3	4	5	6	7	8	9		Average differences								
												1	2	3	4	5	6	7	8	9
55	7404	7412	7419	7427	7435	7443	7451	7459	7466	7474		1	2	2	3	4	5	5	6	7
56	7482	7490	7497	7505	7513	7520	7528	7536	7543	7551		1	2	2	3	4	5	5	6	7
57	7559	7566	7574	7582	7589	7597	7604	7612	7619	7627		1	2	2	3	4	5	5	6	7
58	7634	7642	7649	7657	7664	7672	7679	7686	7694	7701		1	1	2	3	4	4	5	6	7
59	7709	7716	7723	7731	7738	7745	7752	7760	7767	7774		1	1	2	3	4	4	5	6	7
60	7782	7789	7796	7803	7810	7818	7825	7832	7839	7846		1	1	2	3	4	4	5	6	6
61	7853	7860	7868	7875	7882	7889	7896	7903	7910	7917		1	1	2	3	4	4	5	6	6
62	7924	7931	7938	7945	7952	7959	7966	7973	7980	7987		1	1	2	3	3	4	5	6	6
63	7993	8000	8007	8014	8021	8028	8035	8041	8048	8055		1	1	2	3	3	4	5	5	6
64	8062	8069	8075	8082	8089	8096	8102	8109	8116	8122		1	1	2	3	3	4	5	5	6
65	8129	8136	8142	8149	8156	8162	8169	8176	8182	8189		1	1	2	3	3	4	5	5	6
66	8195	8202	8209	8215	8222	8228	8235	8241	8248	8254		1	1	2	3	3	4	5	5	6
67	8261	8267	8274	8280	8287	8293	8299	8306	8312	8319		1	1	2	3	3	4	5	5	6
68	8325	8331	8338	8344	8351	8357	8363	8370	8376	8382		1	1	2	3	3	4	4	5	6
69	8388	8395	8401	8407	8414	8420	8426	8432	8439	8445		1	1	2	2	3	4	4	5	6
70	8451	8457	8463	8470	8476	8482	8488	8494	8500	8506		1	1	2	2	3	4	4	5	6
71	8513	8519	8525	8531	8537	8543	8549	8555	8561	8567		1	1	2	2	3	4	4	5	5
72	8573	8579	8585	8591	8597	8603	8609	8615	8621	8627		1	1	2	2	3	4	4	5	5
73	8633	8639	8645	8651	8657	8663	8669	8675	8681	8686		1	1	2	2	3	4	4	5	5
74	8692	8698	8704	8710	8716	8722	8727	8733	8739	8745		1	1	2	2	3	4	4	5	5
75	8751	8756	8762	8768	8774	8779	8785	8791	8797	8802		1	1	2	2	3	3	4	5	5
76	8808	8814	8820	8825	8831	8837	8842	8848	8854	8859		1	1	2	2	3	3	4	5	5
77	8865	8871	8876	8882	8887	8893	8899	8904	8910	8915		1	1	2	2	3	3	4	4	5
78	8921	8927	8932	8938	8943	8949	8954	8960	8965	8971		1	1	2	2	3	3	4	4	5
79	8976	8982	8987	8993	8998	9004	9009	9015	9020	9025		1	1	2	2	3	3	4	4	5
80	9031	9036	9042	9047	9053	9058	9063	9069	9074	9079		1	1	2	2	3	3	4	4	5
81	9085	9090	9096	9101	9106	9112	9117	9122	9128	9133		1	1	2	2	3	3	4	4	5
82	9138	9143	9149	9154	9159	9165	9170	9175	9180	9186		1	1	2	2	3	3	4	4	5
83	9191	9196	9201	9206	9212	9217	9222	9227	9232	9238		1	1	2	2	3	3	4	4	5
84	9243	9248	9253	9258	9263	9269	9274	9279	9284	9289		1	1	2	2	3	3	4	4	5
85	9294	9299	9304	9309	9315	9320	9325	9330	9335	9340		1	1	2	2	3	3	4	4	5
86	9345	9350	9355	9360	9365	9370	9375	9380	9385	9390		1	1	2	2	3	3	4	4	5
87	9395	9400	9405	9410	9415	9420	9425	9430	9435	9440		0	1	1	2	2	3	3	4	4
88	9445	9450	9455	9460	9465	9469	9474	9484	9489		0	1	1	2	2	3	3	4	4
89	9494	9499	9504	9509	9513	9518	9523	9528	9533	9538		0	1	1	2	2	3	3	4	4
90	9542	9547	9552	9557	9562	9566	9571	9576	9581	9586		0	1	1	2	2	3	3	4	4
91	9590	9595	9600	9605	9609	9614	9619	9624	9628	9633		0	1	1	2	2	3	3	4	4
92	9638	9643	9647	9652	9657	9661	9666	9671	9675	9680		0	1	1	2	2	3	3	4	4
93	9685	9689	9694	9699	9703	9708	9713	9717	9722	9727		0	1	1	2	2	3	3	4	4
94	9731	9736	9741	9745	9750	9754	9759	9763	9768	9773		0	1	1	2	2	3	3	4	4
95	9777	9782	9786	9791	9795	9800	9805	9809	9814	9818		0	1	1	2	2	3	3	4	4
96	9823	9827	9832	9836	9841	9845	9850	9854	9859	9863		0	1	1	2	2	3	3	4	4
97	9868	9872	9877	9881	9886	9890	9894	9899	9903	9908		0	1	1	2	2	3	3	4	4
98	9912	9917	9921	9926	9930	9934	9939	9943	9948	9952		0	1	1	2	2	3	3	4	4
99	9956	9961	9965	9969	9974	9978	9983	9987	9991	9996		0	1	1	2	2	3	3	3	4
x	0	1	2	3	4	5	6	7	8	9		1	2	3	4	5	6	7	8	9

*From Stevenson, R.: Saunders Short Tables, Philadelphia, W. B. Saunders Company, 1967.

ANTILOGARITHMS*

y	0	1	2	3	4	5	6	7	8	9	1	2	3	4	5	6	7	8	9
															Average differences				
0.00	1000	1002	1005	1007	1009	1012	1014	1016	1019	1021	0	0	1	1	1	1	2	2	2
0.01	1023	1026	1028	1030	1033	1035	1038	1040	1042	1045	0	0	1	1	1	1	2	2	2
0.02	1047	1050	1052	1054	1057	1059	1062	1064	1067	1069	0	0	1	1	1	1	2	2	2
0.03	1072	1074	1076	1079	1081	1084	1086	1089	1091	1094	0	0	1	1	1	1	2	2	2
0.04	1096	1099	1102	1104	1107	1109	1112	1114	1117	1119	0	1	1	1	1	2	2	2	2
0.05	1122	1125	1127	1130	1132	1135	1138	1140	1143	1146	0	1	1	1	1	2	2	2	2
0.06	1148	1151	1153	1156	1159	1161	1164	1167	1169	1172	0	1	1	1	1	2	2	2	2
0.07	1175	1178	1180	1183	1186	1189	1191	1194	1197	1199	0	1	1	1	1	2	2	2	2
0.08	1202	1205	1208	1211	1213	1216	1219	1222	1225	1227	0	1	1	1	1	2	2	2	3
0.09	1230	1233	1236	1239	1242	1245	1247	1250	1253	1256	0	1	1	1	1	2	2	2	3
0.10	1259	1262	1265	1268	1271	1274	1276	1279	1282	1285	0	1	1	1	1	2	2	2	3
0.11	1288	1291	1294	1297	1300	1303	1306	1309	1312	1315	0	1	1	1	2	2	2	2	3
0.12	1318	1321	1324	1327	1330	1334	1337	1340	1343	1346	0	1	1	1	2	2	2	2	3
0.13	1349	1352	1355	1358	1361	1365	1368	1371	1374	1377	0	1	1	1	2	2	2	3	3
0.14	1380	1384	1387	1390	1393	1396	1400	1403	1406	1409	0	1	1	1	2	2	2	3	3
0.15	1413	1416	1419	1422	1426	1429	1432	1435	1439	1442	0	1	1	1	2	2	2	3	3
0.16	1445	1449	1452	1455	1459	1462	1466	1469	1472	1476	0	1	1	1	2	2	2	3	3
0.17	1479	1483	1486	1489	1493	1496	1500	1503	1507	1510	0	1	1	1	2	2	2	3	3
0.18	1514	1517	1521	1524	1528	1531	1535	1538	1542	1545	0	1	1	1	2	2	2	3	3
0.19	1549	1552	1556	1560	1563	1567	1570	1574	1578	1581	0	1	1	1	2	2	3	3	3
0.20	1585	1589	1592	1596	1600	1603	1607	1611	1614	1618	0	1	1	1	2	2	3	3	3
0.21	1622	1626	1629	1633	1637	1641	1644	1648	1652	1656	0	1	1	2	2	2	3	3	3
0.22	1660	1663	1667	1671	1675	1679	1683	1687	1690	1694	0	1	1	2	2	2	3	3	3
0.23	1698	1702	1706	1710	1714	1718	1722	1726	1730	1734	0	1	1	2	2	2	3	3	4
0.24	1738	1742	1746	1750	1754	1758	1762	1766	1770	1774	0	1	1	2	2	2	3	3	4
0.25	1778	1782	1786	1791	1795	1799	1803	1807	1811	1816	0	1	1	2	2	2	3	3	4
0.26	1820	1824	1828	1832	1837	1841	1845	1849	1854	1858	0	1	1	2	2	3	3	3	4
0.27	1862	1866	1871	1875	1879	1884	1888	1892	1897	1901	0	1	1	2	2	3	3	3	4
0.28	1905	1910	1914	1919	1923	1928	1932	1936	1941	1945	0	1	1	2	2	3	3	4	4
0.29	1950	1954	1959	1963	1968	1972	1977	1982	1986	1991	0	1	1	2	2	3	3	4	4
0.30	1995	2000	2004	2009	2014	2018	2023	2028	2032	2037	0	1	1	2	2	3	3	4	4
0.31	2042	2046	2051	2056	2061	2065	2070	2075	2080	2084	0	1	1	2	2	3	3	4	4
0.32	2089	2094	2099	2104	2109	2113	2118	2123	2128	2133	0	1	1	2	2	3	3	4	4
0.33	2138	2143	2148	2153	2158	2163	2168	2173	2178	2183	0	1	1	2	2	3	3	4	4
0.34	2188	2193	2198	2203	2208	2213	2218	2223	2228	2234	1	1	2	2	3	3	4	4	5
0.35	2239	2244	2249	2254	2259	2265	2270	2275	2280	2286	1	1	2	2	3	3	4	4	5
0.36	2291	2296	2301	2307	2312	2317	2323	2328	2333	2339	1	1	2	2	3	3	4	4	5
0.37	2344	2350	2355	2360	2366	2371	2377	2382	2388	2393	1	1	2	2	3	3	4	4	5
0.38	2399	2404	2410	2415	2421	2427	2432	2438	2443	2449	1	1	2	2	3	3	4	4	5
0.39	2455	2460	2466	2472	2477	2483	2489	2495	2500	2506	1	1	2	2	3	3	4	5	5
0.40	2512	2518	2523	2529	2535	2541	2547	2553	2559	2564	1	1	2	2	3	4	4	5	5
0.41	2570	2576	2582	2588	2594	2600	2606	2612	2618	2624	1	1	2	2	3	4	4	5	5
0.42	2630	2636	2642	2649	2655	2661	2667	2673	2679	2685	1	1	2	2	3	4	4	5	6
0.43	2692	2698	2704	2710	2716	2723	2729	2735	2742	2748	1	1	2	3	3	4	4	5	6
0.44	2754	2761	2767	2773	2780	2786	2793	2799	2805	2812	1	1	2	3	3	4	4	5	6
0.45	2818	2825	2831	2838	2844	2851	2858	2864	2871	2877	1	1	2	3	3	4	5	5	6
0.46	2884	2891	2897	2904	2911	2917	2924	2931	2938	2944	1	1	2	3	.3	4	5	5	6
0.47	2951	2958	2965	2972	2979	2985	2992	2999	3006	3013	1	1	2	3	3	4	5	5	6
0.48	3020	3027	3034	3041	3048	3055	3062	3069	3076	3083	1	1	2	3	4	4	5	6	6
0.49	3090	3097	3105	3112	3119	3126	3133	3141	3148	3155	1	1	2	3	4	4	5	6	6
	0	1	2	3	4	5	6	7	8	9	1	2	3	4	5	6	7	8	9

*From Stevenson, R.: Saunders Short Tables, Philadelphia, W. B. Saunders Company, 1967.

ANTILOGARITHMS*

y	0	1	2	3	4	5	6	7	8	9	Average differences								
											1	2	3	4	5	6	7	8	9
0.50	3162	3170	3177	3184	3192	3199	3206	3214	3221	3228	1	1	2	3	4	4	5	6	7
0.51	3236	3243	3251	3258	3266	3273	3281	3289	3296	3304	1	2	2	3	4	5	5	6	7
0.52	3311	3319	3327	3334	3342	3350	3357	3365	3373	3381	1	2	2	3	4	5	5	6	7
0.53	3388	3396	3404	3412	3420	3428	3436	3443	3451	3459	1	2	2	3	4	5	6	6	7
0.54	3467	3475	3483	3491	3499	3508	3516	3524	3532	3540	1	2	2	3	4	5	6	6	7
0.55	3548	3556	3565	3573	3581	3589	3597	3606	3614	3622	1	2	2	3	4	5	6	7	7
0.56	3631	3639	3648	3656	3664	3673	3681	3690	3698	3707	1	2	3	3	4	5	6	7	8
0.57	3715	3724	3733	3741	3750	3758	3767	3776	3784	3793	1	2	3	3	4	5	6	7	8
0.58	3802	3811	3819	3828	3837	3846	3855	3864	3873	3882	1	2	3	4	4	5	6	7	8
0.59	3890	3899	3908	3917	3926	3936	3945	3954	3963	3972	1	2	3	4	5	5	6	7	8
0.60	3981	3990	3999	4009	4018	4027	4036	4046	4055	4064	1	2	3	4	5	6	6	7	8
0.61	4074	4083	4093	4102	4111	4121	4130	4140	4150	4159	1	2	3	4	5	6	7	8	9
0.62	4169	4178	4188	4198	4207	4217	4227	4236	4246	4256	1	2	3	4	5	6	7	8	9
0.63	4266	4276	4285	4295	4305	4315	4325	4335	4345	4355	1	2	3	4	5	6	7	8	9
0.64	4365	4375	4385	4395	4406	4416	4426	4436	4446	4457	1	2	3	4	5	6	7	8	9
0.65	4467	4477	4487	4498	4508	4519	4529	4539	4550	4560	1	2	3	4	5	6	7	8	9
0.66	4571	4581	4592	4603	4613	4624	4634	4645	4656	4667	1	2	3	4	5	6	7	9	10
0.67	4677	4688	4699	4710	4721	4732	4742	4753	4764	4775	1	2	3	4	5	7	8	9	10
0.68	4786	4797	4808	4819	4831	4842	4853	4864	4875	4887	1	2	3	4	6	7	8	9	10
0.69	4898	4909	4920	4932	4943	4955	4966	4977	4989	5000	1	2	3	5	6	7	8	9	10
0.70	5012	5023	5035	5047	5058	5070	5082	5093	5105	5117	1	2	4	5	6	7	8	9	11
0.71	5129	5140	5152	5164	5176	5188	5200	5212	5224	5236	1	2	4	5	6	7	8	10	11
0.72	5248	5260	5272	5284	5297	5309	5321	5333	5346	5358	1	2	4	5	6	7	9	10	11
0.73	5370	5383	5395	5408	5420	5433	5445	5458	5470	5483	1	3	4	5	6	8	9	10	11
0.74	5495	5508	5521	5534	5546	5559	5572	5585	5598	5610	1	3	4	5	6	8	9	10	12
0.75	5623	5636	5649	5662	5675	5689	5702	5715	5728	5741	1	3	4	5	7	8	9	10	12
0.76	5754	5768	5781	5794	5808	5821	5834	5848	5861	5875	1	3	4	5	7	8	9	11	12
0.77	5888	5902	5916	5929	5943	5957	5970	5984	5998	6012	1	3	4	5	7	8	10	11	12
0.78	6026	6039	6053	6067	6081	6095	6109	6124	6138	6152	1	3	4	6	7	8	10	11	13
0.79	6166	6180	6194	6209	6223	6237	6252	6266	6281	6295	1	3	4	6	7	9	10	11	13
0.80	6310	6324	6339	6353	6368	6383	6397	6412	6427	6442	1	3	4	6	7	9	10	12	13
0.81	6457	6471	6486	6501	6516	6531	6546	6561	6577	6592	2	3	5	6	8	9	11	12	14
0.82	6607	6622	6637	6653	6668	6683	6699	6714	6730	6745	2	3	5	6	8	9	11	12	14
0.83	6761	6776	6792	6808	6823	6839	6855	6871	6887	6902	2	3	5	6	8	9	11	13	14
0.84	6918	6934	6950	6966	6982	6998	7015	7031	7047	7063	2	3	5	6	8	10	11	13	15
0.85	7079	7096	7112	7129	7145	7161	7178	7194	7211	7228	2	3	5	7	8	10	12	13	15
0.86	7244	7261	7278	7295	7311	7328	7345	7362	7379	7396	2	3	5	7	8	10	12	13	15
0.87	7413	7430	7447	7464	7482	7499	7516	7534	7551	7568	2	3	5	7	9	10	12	14	16
0.88	7586	7603	7621	7638	7656	7674	7691	7709	7727	7745	2	4	5	7	9	11	12	14	16
0.89	7762	7780	7798	7816	7834	7852	7870	7889	7907	7925	2	4	5	7	9	11	13	14	16
0.90	7943	7962	7980	7998	8017	8035	8054	8072	8091	8110	2	4	6	7	9	11	13	15	17
0.91	8128	8147	8166	8185	8204	8222	8241	8260	8279	8299	2	4	6	8	9	11	13	15	17
0.92	8318	8337	8356	8375	8395	8414	8433	8453	8472	8492	2	4	6	8	10	12	14	15	17
0.93	8511	8531	8551	8570	8590	8610	8630	8650	8670	8690	2	4	6	8	10	12	14	16	18
0.94	8710	8730	8750	8770	8790	8810	8831	8851	8872	8892	2	4	6	8	10	12	14	16	18
0.95	8913	8933	8954	8974	8995	9016	9036	9057	9078	9099	2	4	6	8	10	12	15	17	19
0.96	9120	9141	9162	9183	9204	9226	9247	9268	9290	9311	2	4	6	8	11	13	15	17	19
0.97	9333	9354	9376	9397	9419	9441	9462	9484	9506	9528	2	4	7	9	11	13	15	17	20
0.98	9550	9572	9594	9616	9638	9661	9683	9705	9727	9750	2	4	7	9	11	13	16	18	20
0.99	9772	9795	9817	9840	9863	9886	9908	9931	9954	9977	2	5	7	9	11	14	16	18	20
	0	1	2	3	4	5	6	7	8	9	1	2	3	4	5	6	7	8	9

*From Stevenson, R.: Saunders Short Tables, Philadelphia, W. B. Saunders Company, 1967.

% TRANSMISSION – ABSORBANCE
CONVERSION CHART

% T	A	% T	A	% T	A	% T	A
1	2.000	1.5	1.824	51	.2924	51.5	.2882
2	1.699	2.5	1.602	52	.2840	52.5	.2798
3	1.523	3.5	1.456	53	.2756	53.5	.2716
4	1.398	4.5	1.347	54	.2676	54.5	.2636
5	1.301	5.5	1.260	55	.2596	55.5	.2557
6	1.222	6.5	1.187	56	.2518	56.5	.2480
7	1.155	7.5	1.126	57	.2441	57.5	.2403
8	1.097	8.5	1.071	58	.2366	58.5	.2328
9	1.046	9.5	1.022	59	.2291	59.5	.2255
10	1.000	10.5	.979	60	.2218	60.5	.2182
11	.959	11.5	.939	61	.2147	61.5	.2111
12	.921	12.5	.903	62	.2076	62.5	.2041
13	.886	13.5	.870	63	.2007	63.5	.1973
14	.854	14.5	.838	64	.1939	64.5	.1905
15	.824	15.5	.810	65	.1871	65.5	.1838
16	.796	16.5	.782	66	.1805	66.5	.1772
17	.770	17.5	.757	67	.1739	67.5	.1707
18	.745	18.5	.733	68	.1675	68.5	.1643
19	.721	19.5	.710	69	.1612	69.5	.1580
20	.699	20.5	.688	70	.1549	70.5	.1518
21	.678	21.5	.668	71	.1487	71.5	.1457
22	.658	22.5	.648	72	.1427	72.5	.1397
23	.638	23.5	.629	73	.1367	73.5	.1337
24	.620	24.5	.611	74	.1308	74.5	.1278
25	.602	25.5	.594	75	.1249	75.5	.1221
26	.585	26.5	.577	76	.1192	76.5	.1163
27	.569	27.5	.561	77	.1135	77.5	.1107
28	.553	28.5	.545	78	.1079	78.5	.1051
29	.538	29.5	.530	79	.1024	79.5	.0996
30	.523	30.5	.516	80	.0969	80.5	.0942
31	.509	31.5	.502	81	.0915	81.5	.0888
32	.495	32.5	.488	82	.0862	82.5	.0835
33	.482	33.5	.475	83	.0809	83.5	.0783
34	.469	34.5	.462	84	.0757	84.5	.0731
35	.456	35.5	.450	85	.0706	85.5	.0680
36	.444	36.5	.438	86	.0655	86.5	.0630
37	.432	37.5	.426	87	.0605	87.5	.0580
38	.420	38.5	.414	88	.0555	88.5	.0531
39	.409	39.5	.403	89	.0505	89.5	.0482
40	.398	40.5	.392	90	.0458	90.5	.0434
41	.387	41.5	.382	91	.0410	91.5	.0386
42	.377	42.5	.372	92	.0362	92.5	.0339
43	.367	43.5	.362	93	.0315	93.5	.0292
44	.357	44.5	.352	94	.0269	94.5	.0246
45	.347	45.5	.342	95	.0223	95.5	.0200
46	.337	46.5	.332	96	.0177	96.5	.0155
47	.328	47.5	.323	97	.0132	97.5	.0110
48	.319	48.5	.314	98	.0088	98.5	.0066
49	.310	49.5	.305	99	.0044	99.5	.0022
50	.301	50.5	.297	100	.0000		.0000

TABLE OF ATOMIC WEIGHTS
(Based on Carbon-12)

	Symbol	Atomic No.	Atomic Weight		Symbol	Atomic No.	Atomic Weight
Actinium	Ac	89	227	Mercury	Hg	80	200.59
Aluminum	Al	13	26.9815	Molybdenum	Mo	42	95.94
Americium	Am	95	[243]*	Neodymium	Nd	60	144.24
Antimony	Sb	51	121.75	Neon	Ne	10	20.183
Argon	Ar	18	39.948	Neptunium	Np	93	[237]
Arsenic	As	33	74.9216	Nickel	Ni	28	58.71
Astatine	At	85	[210]	Niobium	Nb	41	92.906
Barium	Ba	56	137.34	Nitrogen	N	7	14.0067
Berkelium	Bk	97	[249]	Nobelium	No	102	[253]
Beryllium	Be	4	9.0122	Osmium	Os	76	190.2
Bismuth	Bi	83	208.980	Oxygen	O	8	15.9994
Boron	B	5	10.811	Palladium	Pd	46	106.4
Bromine	Br	35	79.909	Phosphorus	P	15	30.9738
Cadmium	Cd	48	112.40	Platinum	Pt	78	195.09
Calcium	Ca	20	40.08	Plutonium	Pu	94	[242]
Californium	Cf	98	[251]	Polonium	Po	84	210
Carbon	C	6	12.01115	Potassium	K	19	39.102
Cerium	Ce	58	140.12	Praseodymium	Pr	59	140.907
Cesium	Cs	55	132.905	Promethium	Pm	61	[145]
Chlorine	Cl	17	35.453	Protactinium	Pa	91	231
Chromium	Cr	24	51.996	Radium	Ra	88	226.05
Cobalt	Co	27	58.9332	Radon	Rn	86	222
Copper	Cu	29	63.54	Rhenium	Re	75	186.2
Curium	Cm	96	[247]	Rhodium	Rh	45	102.905
Dysprosium	Dy	66	162.50	Rubidium	Rb	37	85.47
Einsteinium	Es	99	[254]	Ruthenium	Ru	44	101.07
Erbium	Er	68	167.26	Samarium	Sm	62	150.35
Europium	Eu	63	151.96	Scandium	Sc	21	44.956
Fermium	Fm	100	[253]	Selenium	Se	34	78.96
Fluorine	F	9	18.9984	Silicon	Si	14	28.086
Francium	Fr	87	[223]	Silver	Ag	47	107.870
Gadolinium	Gd	64	157.25	Sodium	Na	11	22.9898
Gallium	Ga	31	69.72	Strontium	Sr	38	87.62
Germanium	Ge	32	72.59	Sulfur	S	16	32.064
Gold	Au	79	196.967	Tantalum	Ta	73	180.948
Hafnium	Hf	72	178.49	Technetium	Tc	43	[99]
Helium	He	2	4.0026	Tellurium	Te	52	127.60
Holmium	Ho	67	164.930	Terbium	Tb	65	158.924
Hydrogen	H	1	1.00797	Thallium	Tl	81	204.37
Indium	In	49	114.82	Thorium	Th	90	232.038
Iodine	I	53	126.9044	Thulium	Tm	69	168.934
Iridium	Ir	77	192.2	Tin	Sn	50	118.69
Iron	Fe	26	55.847	Titanium	Ti	22	47.90
Krypton	Kr	36	83.80	Tungsten	W	74	183.85
Lanthanum	La	57	138.91	Uranium	U	92	238.03
Lawrencium	Lw	103	[257]	Vanadium	V	23	50.942
Lead	Pb	82	207.19	Xenon	Xe	54	131.30
Lithium	Li	3	6.939	Ytterbium	Yb	70	173.04
Lutetium	Lu	71	174.97	Yttrium	Y	39	88.905
Magnesium	Mg	12	24.312	Zinc	Zn	30	65.37
Manganese	Mn	25	54.9380	Zirconium	Zr	40	91.22
Mendelevium	Md	101	[256]				

*A value given in brackets denotes the mass number of the longest-lived or best-known isotope.

CONCENTRATED SOLUTIONS OF ACIDS AND BASES

Acid or Base	Molecular Weight	Specific Gravity	% by Weight	Approx. Normality	Approx. ml/l for 1 N soln.
Acetic acid CH_3COOH	60	1.06	99.5	17	59
Hydrochloric acid, HCl	36.5	1.19	37	12	83
Nitric acid, HNO_3	63	1.42	70	16	63
Phosphoric acid, H_3PO_4	98	1.71	87	45	25
Sulfuric acid, H_2SO_4	98	1.84	96	36	28
Ammonium hydroxide, NH_4OH	35	0.88	29	16	63
Potassium hydroxide, KOH (satd. soln.)	56.1	1.55	about 50	14	71
Sodium hydroxide, NaOH (satd. soln.)	40	1.52	about 50	17	60

Nomogram for calculating the total CO_2, $HCO_3{}^-$, pH, Pco_2 or $HHCO_3$. A straight line is drawn between the two known points and the desired value is read from the other two scales. Example: the total CO_2 and the pH are known and their values are 13 and 7.2, respectively. If we draw a line through these two points we will find a Pco_2 value of 31 mm. Hg, an $HHCO_3$ value of 0.93 and an $HCO_3{}^-$value of 12.1. All values are only approximate. (From Van Slyke D. D. and Sendroy, J. Biol. Chem., 79: 781, 1928. Reproduced with the permission of the author and The American Society of Biological Chemists, Inc.)

NOMOGRAM FOR THE DETERMINATON OF
BODY SURFACE AREA OF CHILDREN*

Weight (Mass†)

Pounds   Kilograms

Body Surface
in square meters

Height
Feet and inches   Centimeters

*From DuBois, E. F.: *Basal Metabolism in Health and Disease.* Philadelphia, Lea & Febiger, 1936.

NOMOGRAM FOR THE DETERMINATION OF BODY SURFACE OF CHILDREN AND ADULTS*

*From Boothby, W. M., and Sandiford, R. B.: Boston M. & S.J. *185*:337, 1921.

IODINE-125 DECAY TABLE
HALF-LIFE: 60 DAYS

	0	2	4	6	8	10	12	14	16	18
0	–	.977	.955	.933	.912	.891	.871	.851	.831	.812
20	.794	.778	.758	.741	.724	.707	.691	.675	.660	.645
40	.630	.616	.602	.588	.574	.561	.548	.536	.524	.512
60	.500	.489	.477	.467	.456	.445	.435	.425	.416	.406
80	.397	.388	.379	.370	.362	.354	.345	.338	.330	.322
100	.315	.308	.301	.294	.287	.281	.274	.268	.262	.256
120	.250	.244	.239	.233	.228	.223	.218	.213	.208	.203

Days (column header), Days (row label)

TABLE*

$n' \dagger$	50%	95%	99%
1	1.000	12.706	63.657
2	.816	4.303	9.925
3	.765	3.182	5.841
4	.741	2.776	4.604
5	.727	2.571	4.032
6	.718	2.447	3.707
7	.711	2.365	3.499
8	.706	2.306	3.355
9	.703	2.262	3.250
10	.700	2.228	3.169
11	.697	2.201	3.106
12	.695	2.179	3.055
13	.694	2.160	3.012
14	.692	2.145	2.977
15	.691	2.131	2.947
16	.690	2.120	2.921
17	.689	2.110	2.898
18	.688	2.101	2.878
19	.688	2.093	2.861
20	.687	2.086	2.845
21	.686	2.080	2.831
22	.686	2.074	2.819
23	.685	2.069	2.807
24	.685	2.064	2.797
25	.684	2.060	2.787
26	.684	2.056	2.779
27	.684	2.052	2.771
28	.683	2.048	2.763
29	.683	2.045	2.756
30	.683	2.042	2.750

*This table is generally referred to as the t table and the value in the body of the table as t. It is to be used only when the standard deviation of the universe is estimated by using the sample standard deviation in the standard error formula.

†The n' in the table represents the degrees of freedom. For the standard error of the mean this is $n - 1$.

ANSWERS TO EXERCISES

Chapter 1

Section 1.2

A. $2\frac{1}{12}$ F. 1.325   J. 30

B. $3\frac{1}{6}$ G. 16.4   K. 0.01

C. $8\frac{3}{4}$ H. 22.54   L. 10^{-3}

D. $2\frac{7}{16}$ I. 3.35   M. 200

E. $7\frac{7}{24}$

Additional Exercises

1. $0.35   b. 600   e. 4.4×10^{-7}
2. $100,000   c. 5   f. 5.0×10^{-9}
3. 104°F.   7a. 2.2×10^6 8a. 9.43×10^9
4. -112°F.   b. 4.6×10^4 b. 4.032×10^{12}
5. 21.1°C   c. 1.51×10^5 c. 6.82×10^{-9}
6a. 1500   d. 3.0×10^{-4} d. 27

Chapter 2

Section 2.3
A. 0.7404   C. $\overline{2}.7924$ or $8.7924 - 10$ E. $\overline{1}.1761$ or $9.1761 - 10$
B. 2.6345   D. 3.5110

Section 2.4
A. 20.78   C. 1.847   E. 0.2327
B. 1515.5   D. 0.03774

Section 2.5
A. 19.7   B. 317.8   C. 0.0032

Section 2.6
A. 4.84   B. 33.25   C. 503.9

Section 2.9

A. 602,180
B. 43,240

C. 9.28
D. 6.8573

E. log 7.7160 - 10

Additional Exercises

1a. 2
 b. $\overline{2}$ or 8 - 10
 c. $\overline{5}$ or 5 - 10
 d. 1
 e. 0
4a. 604
 b. 3.970
 c. 0.02780
 d. 97.21
 e. 0.00428

2a. 0.6628
 b. 0.6628
 c. 0.8921
 d. 0.1553
 e. 0.8451
5a. 2310
 b. 9408
 c. 29217
 d. 118.5
 e. 1.054

3a. 2.8274
 b. 0.1761
 c. 4.5315
 d. 3.5315 or 7.5315 - 10
6a. 5415
 b. 2.132
 c. 3.484
 d. 5.9085
 e. $\overline{6}$.3802 or 4.3802 - 10

Chapter 3

Section 3.2

A. 585
B. 735

C. 630
D. 130

Section 3.4

A. 56.1
B. 53,250

C. 52,250
D. 12.68

E. 2.66

Section 3.5

A. 8.82

B. 2350

C. 221

Section 3.6

A. 11.68
B. 78.1

C. 4.49
D. 187,400

E. 18.66

Section 3.7

A. 13.45
B. 492
C. 48.7
D. 666,000

E. 8.12
F. 23.8
G. 0.2085
H. 2.55

I. 0.01298
J. 71.6

Section 3.8

A. 59.7 cm
B. 4.57 m
C. 8.87 ml
D. 324.0 mg

E. 54.5 kg
F. 110 lb
G. 12.88 km
H. X = 11.12

I. X = 0.75
J. X = 30

Section 3.9

A. 826
B. 630
C. 75.8
D. 52,200
E. 11.5

F. 1680
G. 27.5
H. 46.5
I. 8.54
J. 0.0667

K. 154 lb
L. X = 38
M. 241.3 km

Additional Exercises

1a. 2860	2a. 1760	3a. 980	4a. 358 cm	5a. X = 40
b. 227.8	b. 67.5	b. 2.28	b. 91.44 cm	b. 110.1 lb
c. 9220	c. 114.4	c. 23.5	c. 90.9 kg	c. 7.71 gr
d. 297,300	d. 22.46	d. 0.2368	d. 59.1 kg	d. 8800 yd
e. 1,400,000	e. 570.5	e. 8.215	e. 648 mg	e. 33.82 oz
			f. 81 mg	
			g. 96.6 km	
			h. 236.6 ml	

Chapter 4

Section 4.2

A. 57.5 g   B. 123.5 g

Section 4.3

A. 12.9 liters   B. 13.6   C. 4.46 g

Section 4.4

A. 62.5%   B. 108.5 g

Section 4.5

A. 60 g   B. 17.55 µg   C. 100 mM

Section 4.7

A. 16.3 ml   B. 0.145 N   C. 5 liters

Section 4.8

A. 200 ml   C. 45 ml   E. 600 mg/dl
B. 825 ml   D. 10 mg/dl

Section 4.9

A. 109.5 ml   Bb. 36.8 N   Bc. 12.5 N
Ba. 12.2 N

Additional Exercises

1. 50 g
2. 1.020
3. 99.2 g
4. Anhydrous

5. 0.098 g
6. 46.8 g
7. 2.72 ml
8. 592 ml

9. 266.7 ml
10. 29.2%
11. 250 ml
12. 104.1 mEq/1

Chapter 5

Exercises

1. 0.0003
2. 0.095
3. 1×10^{-4} ; 4

4. 3.4
5. 0.014; 1.8; 1.85

6. 7.51
7. 3.16×10^{-4}

Chapter 6

Exercises

A. pH 7.10
B. pH 5.73

C. pK_a 6.10

D. From pH 4.73
   to pH 4.69

Additional Exercises

1. pH 7.23
2. 44.5 mm Hg
3. 41.2 mm Hg

4. 25.8 mM/l
5. pH 7.55
6. 25.2 mM/l

7. 25.4 mM/l
8. 36.7 mm Hg

Chapter 7

Exercises

1. 54.2 ml/min; 72.3%
2. 15 ml/min; 27.8%
3. 107.2 ml/min

4. 0.397 square meters
5. 111.3 ml/min

6. 140.1 ml/min
7. 72.3 ml/min

Chapter 8

A. 4250

B. 1.085

Additional Exercises

1. 17,300
2. 0.545

3. 38.5 mg/dl

4. 1.2 mg/dl

5.

No, Beer's law is not followed at the two highest concentrations. Slight variation at 4 mg/dl, considerable at 5.

6.   a. 4.32 mg/dl   c. 3.30 mg/dl
       b. 3.38 mg/dl   d. 4.46 mg/dl

7.

7a. 125.6 mEq/l
 b. 141.2 mEq/l
 c. 134.4 mEq/l
 d. 135.8 mEq/l

Chapter 9

Section 9.1
A. 90.0%   C. 7.74 mCi   E. 0.3349/min; 12.8 mCi
B. 3.62 mCi   D. 14.29 d; 108.3 μCi

Section 9.2
A. 25.9%   C. 31.5%
B. 0.277 mm; 28.6%   D. 22.48 mr/h

Section 9.3
A. 26.1 d   B. 33.26 d

Section 9.4
A. 2.026×10^{-8} g; 4.94×10^7 mCi/g   C. Monday, 6:14 P.M.
B. 69.28 μCi/ml

Section 9.5
A. 15 μCi/ml   C. 1.4 ml   E. 7.5 ml
B. 160 μCi/ml   D. 0.167 ml

Chapter 10

1. Both x and y are variables while a and b are constants. As the graph of an equation for a straight line when y is plotted on the ordinate, x on the abscissa; the slope of the line is a and the intercept on the y axis is b.

2. x and y since x is usually plotted as the concentration of a standard solution or as time in hours and y is ordinarily plotted as absorbance readings or as concentration as in glucose tolerance curves.

3.

4.

This is not a satisfactory standard curve since the line does not go through the origin. A common dilution error of the standard solutions used in preparation of the curve is the probable reason for the unsatisfactory curve.

5.

6.

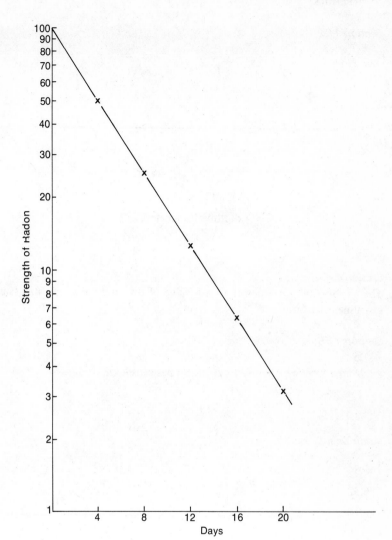

Chapter 11

Section 11.1

A. 1.49 mEq/l

B.   Males $S = 0.216$ C. V. 3.54%

                  Females $S = 0.134$ C. V. 2.34%

Section 11.2

A.

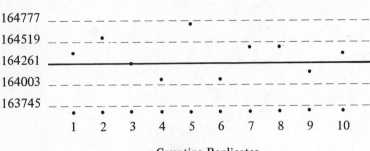

Counting Replicates

Section 11.3

A. The χ^2 of 3.69 corresponds to a p value of over 0.90 and indicates faulty instrument performance.

Section 11.6

A. −4.06

B. −2.98; the t value is significant at the 95 per cent level.

Additional Exercises

1.

6.54																						+2s
6.32								•						•								+1s
6.10		•										•					•				X̄
5.88				• •						•			•								−1s
5.66																						−2s

2.

12.71																	•	+2s
12.52				•		•			•		•				+1s
12.33			•					• •			• •	X̄
12.14	•		• •				•		• •			−1s
11.95		•		•		•				−2s

3.

102.52	+2s
100.76	+1s
99.00	$\overline{X}$
97.24	-1s
95.48	-2s

INDEX